INSPIRED MEDICINE

Sathya Sai Baba's Influence in Medical Practice

Compiled & Edited by Judy Warner

DISTRIBUTED BY
SATHYA SAI BOOK CENTER
OF AMERICA
305 W. FIRST STREET
TUSTIN, CA 92780, USA
714-669-0522

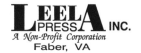
LEELA
PRESS INC.
A Non-Profit Corporation
Faber, VA

English edition first published in 2000 by
Leela Press, Inc.
4026 River Road
Faber, VA 22938

Library of Congress Card Number: 00-103911

Inspired Medicine: Sathya's Sai Baba's Influence in Medical Practice
Compiled and edited by Judy Warner

Cover: Eleni Mylonas

ISBN: 1-887906-02-9

Dedicated with love and devotion
to
Bhagavan Sri Sathya Sai Baba

Other Books by Judy Warner:

Transformation of the Heart
(Stories by Devotees of Sathya Sai Baba)

The Dharmic Challenge
(Putting Sathya Sai Baba's Teachings into Practice)

FOREWORD

In this fascinating book, eighteen physicians from different specialties and backgrounds describe the profound influence Sathya Sai Baba has had on their personal and professional lives. World class doctors, acclaimed in their fields in cardiac surgery, diabetes and gynecology – intelligent, sensitive, articulate men and women, from Thailand, India, Europe, South America, Canada and the U.S., unexpectedly find themselves brought into the sphere of Sai Baba's love. In a delightful unfolding of the impossible, dry hearts are transformed into love and egos humbly bow to God.

Each story takes us into the hectic lives of practicing physicians, revealing their everyday battles with life and death problems. The attraction each one has to Sai Baba is profound. In the face of this tension, how surprising to find such humor and play accompanying their meetings with Sai Baba. Each is deeply impressed by His love and the way His teachings are practiced in His Super Specialty Hospital. Each doctor enters into a searching personal inquiry to make basic changes to his life and profession. We see in the lives of these doctors a happy marriage of medicine and spirituality.

This marvelous book about the inner transformation of the practitioner and the practice of medicine offers a wonderful glimpse into a penetrating new insight taking place in medicine inspired by the divine figure, Sathya Sai Baba. His hospital symbolizes a new approach to medicine in which care is provided free of charge and love is an essential ingredient in the healing process. The stories describe a grand historic event – a world teacher brings heart into a field which has long been tempted by money and position. *Science without humanity is dangerous,* Sai Baba says. This is a book of miracle, marvel and medicine that has the power to amaze, delight, teach and transform.

Samuel H. Sandweiss, M.D.
Sai Baba, The Holy Man and the Psychiatrist
Spirit and the Mind

i

ACKNOWLEDGMENTS

First and foremost, I want to express my gratitude to my Beloved Lord, Sathya Sai Baba; without His will, this book would never have been written.

I want to thank all those who helped me find the doctors to write for *Inspired Medicine*. I also want to thank the doctor/authors for the time, love and energy they gave to this project.

I want to thank Dimitri Drivas and Lola Goldberg for their help with copy editing.

My thanks to Eleni Mylonas for her wonderful cover design and execution, as well as Emily Goodman for her technical support.

My husband had the idea for this book and supported this effort from start to finish. With love and thanks to you, Jack.

TABLE OF CONTENTS

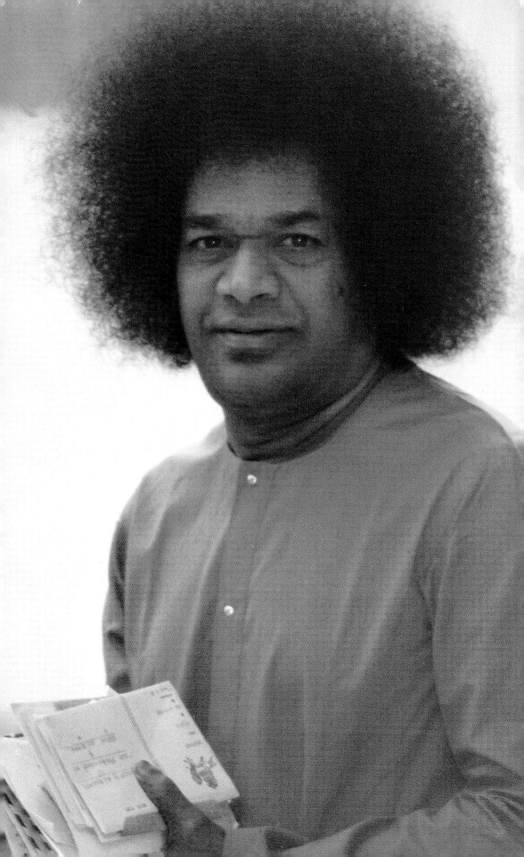

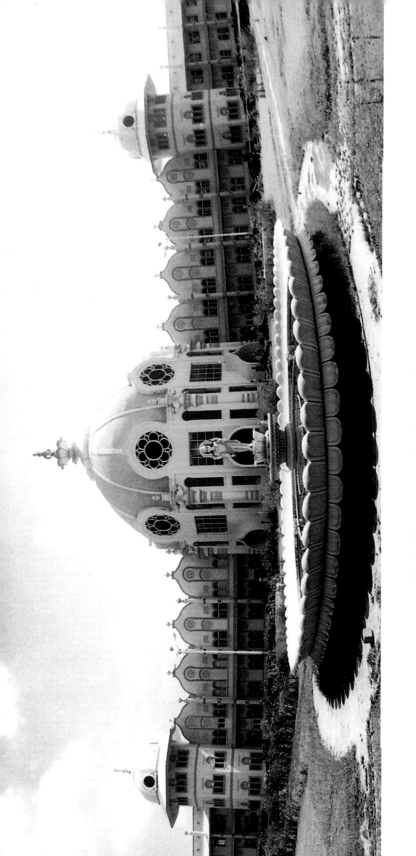

Sri Sathya Sai Institute
of Higher Medical Sciences

About the Super Specialty Hospital

The Sathya Sai Institute of Higher Medical Sciences is located outside the village of Puttaparti in South India. It is a 300-bed facility with state-of-the-art equipment in all its departments: Cardiology, Cardiac Surgery, Urology, Nephrology and Ophthalmology. All services, such as diagnostics, operations, including surgery and anesthesiology, doctor's fees, hospital stay, food and medicine are completely free. Most of the procedures performed are to the very poor. The hospital was built by and runs completely on donations given by the devotees of Sathya Sai Baba. This confirms the hospital's philosophy that the cost of providing medical care should be absorbed by society and not be priced and sold in the market as a commodity. The hospital is open to all citizens of the world irrespective of nationality, caste, creed, language or financial status.

Leading medical specialists from all over the world come and volunteer to donate their services. They complement the hospital's highly competent team of doctors. The visiting physicians perform operations and teach the staff the latest techniques in their field of medicine.

Through February 2000, 9,078 heart operations were performed, over 5,000 on open hearts of which over 1,000 were coronary artery bypass grafts. There were over 8,000 cardiac catheterizations performed, and the Departments of Urology and Ophthalmology each performed over 11,000 operations. The infection and mortality rate experienced is among the lowest in the world.

The hospital's architecture, by design, embodies the symbolism and proportions of sacred traditions that are believed to engender a divine healing energy. This state-of-the-art 15,000 square meter facility was miraculously designed and constructed within nine months. It ranks as the second largest hospital in Asia. A facility of this size usually takes about seven years from inception to completion. The architect was Dr. Keith Critchlow, Director, Prince of Wales Institute of Architecture in London. The Sathya Sai Institute of Higher Medical Sciences was opened and inaugurated by the Prime Minister of India on November 22nd, 1991.

Note:

Italics are used when Sathya Sai Baba is speaking.

There is a glossary of sanskrit words in the back of the book.

INTRODUCTION

Sathya Sai Baba was born in 1926 in the small village of Puttaparthi in southern India, where His ashram now stands. He came into the world with all knowledge, wisdom, power and divine love. He is considered by his followers to be an avatar, a divine incarnation of God. Today, He has over thirty million followers in 137 countries around the world. He teaches the brotherhood of man and the fatherhood of God through the five human values of Truth, Right Action, Peace, Love and Nonviolence. He is the living example of all that He teaches. His mission is to transform humanity to *know* that they, too, are divine.

Throughout the world, physicians are trained to rely solely on scientific principles. Unfortunately, many have lost their compassion and view medical practice as a business. We wondered, what would happen to doctors and their practice once they became devoted to Sai Baba? Eighteen physicians were asked to tell how becoming a Sai devotee influenced the way they practice medicine, how it has changed their relationship with their patients, how they have changed as doctors, how they have felt Sai Baba's hand in their practice, and if they have experienced any miracles.

One of the themes that echo again and again among the physician/authors is the realization that the most important part of a physician's practice is the giving of love and compassion to the patient. Fortunately, we have begun to see recognition of this idea within the Western complementary medical community.

In January 1999, my husband and I presented Baba with an outline for *Inspired Medicine,* and He gave us His blessing to compile and edit this book. As we all know, doctors are extremely busy. But, by Baba's grace, physicians from Asia, Europe, and North and South America have willingly worked and re-worked their stories in order to celebrate their love for the Lord. We presented Swami with the manuscript in March 2000 and asked His permission to publish the book. Smiling, He placed His hand on the cover and said sweetly, "Very, very, very, very happy." May these stories uplift you and bring joy and love to your life.

JW

vii

Believe firmly that the BODY IS THE RESIDENCE OF GOD; that the food you eat is the offering you make to your Deity; that bathing is the ceremonial bathing of the Divine Spirit in you; the ground you walk upon is His domain; the joy you derive is His gift; the grief you experience is His lesson that you tread the path more carefully. Remember Him even in sun and shade, day and night, awake or asleep.

Sathya Sai Baba
Sanathana Sarathi, Vol. 26 #1, November 1983, back page

Sathya Sai Baba, Transplanter of My Heart
Valluvan Jeevanandam, M.D.

My humblest pranams at the lotus feet of my divine mother and father, Bhagavan Sathya Sai Baba. It is with Baba's energy and guidance that I can write this chapter. I am neither a philosopher nor a theologian, and my spiritual abilities certainly need to be developed. What I will relate is how I became a Sai Baba devotee, some Sai incidences I have personally experienced, and how Swami has affected my life and work.

Baba says that He will call us only when it is the proper time. The first time I heard about Swami was in 1980. My aunt took my mother, sister, and me to visit Kodaikanal and insisted that we go to see Baba there. She said He was a holy man who would grant interviews, materialize things, and predict the future. Being a typical American young adult, my concept of every swami was that of a fraudulent cult leader who would try to extract every penny one had. I refused to see this holy man. This was an enormous mistake, but it just wasn't my time. If I had gone, my life would have changed almost a decade earlier. At that time, there were about 200 devotees in Kodaikanal. I could have had close, personal experiences with Baba. But my mind refused to accept anything spiritual at that time.

I spent the subsequent ten years finishing medical school and my residency in cardiac surgery. Religion and spirituality were the last things on my mind. My sole focus was making a lot of money, buying a huge house, driving luxurious cars, and eating at the best restaurants. A life of material wealth was mine for the taking. Swami was just letting me play awhile, for during that period my spiritual path was practically non-existent.

Baba started me on the divine path without my ever realizing it. My parents have always been religious, especially my mother. I have disappointed her many times by not learning slokas and doing daily prayer. My parents moved to Arizona and began attending the Sai Baba center in Mesa. Whenever my family and I visited them, they would take us to Sunday bhajans. That was not exactly what I wanted to do during my short vacations. I would even try to schedule the plane flights to avoid the bhajans. But with my mother's guidance, I started to listen to and actually enjoy bhajan tapes. My interest in Baba was further heightened when I read Howard

Murphet's *Sai Baba: Man of Miracles.* Baba was no longer an entity to run from, but not one to be believed either. Bhajan tapes slowly replaced pop music as the preferred music in the car.

After finishing surgical training, the stresses of being a new attending physician took up most of my time. My mother sent me several Baba books to read, but I always had an excuse not to read them. Miraculously, we found a Baba center in Doylestown, Pennsylvania, which was a mere 15 minutes away, and that's when Baba began drawing us into His net. The most dramatic event occurred in November 1992 during a visit to Arizona for Thanksgiving. I had prepared for the long flight with the usual set of novels and other time-consuming materials. After I got on the plane and opened my bag, none of the reading material I had packed was there. The only book was *The Vision of Sai* by Rita Bruce. Absolutely nothing else! Without any options, I started reading the book, clearly expecting to fall asleep within half an hour. Well, I was never so mesmerized and moved by a book. Swami had finally caught me. I was previously a non-vegetarian who really enjoyed every meat dish possible. I stepped out of the airplane a vegetarian, much to the utter astonishment of my wife and parents. I have remained a pure vegetarian, despite eating at some of the fanciest restaurants in the world. All my previous acquaintances were astonished. I was finally on the divine path toward Swami.

The next big event that catapulted me toward Swami occurred in April 1993. We had a guest speaker at one of our Sunday bhajans who told us about the new Super Specialty Hospital in Puttaparthi where cardiac surgery is done absolutely free. Because I was also a cardiac surgeon, I was introduced to the speaker. During the conversation, he said that the availability of artificial heart valves was limited in India and asked whether there was anything I could do to help. I had absolutely no idea how to proceed further. Valves are very expensive in the United States and, being a new attending physician, the spirit was there in wanting to help, but the wallet was not. This was to become one of Swami's amazing leelas. The next day, I got a call from an old friend from whom I had not heard in a year. It seemed that he had switched jobs and was working for St. Jude Medical, the largest manufacturer of heart valves in the world.

Furthermore, he was in charge of the Asian market. He arranged for me to buy valves at cost and, in addition, arranged for a matching donation from his company. In one telephone call things went from impossible to reality. Later, a representative who sold sutures contacted me. He had a huge overstock of very expensive heart sutures and wanted to know if there were any hospitals doing charity work that could use them. Swami was guiding me through an incredible shopping spree. Finally, it was the middle of May, and I had a lot of equipment but no time off to take it to India. We were short on faculty, and there was no relief in sight. My prayers to Swami were answered when we were finally able to recruit a very good surgeon. However, he wanted three weeks off to visit his family in Japan. Without my asking, my boss came to me with a proposition. Since the new attending physician was taking time off, how about if I took an equal amount of time off in July? I was dumbfounded. Even without asking, I was being given time to visit Puttaparthi. Swami was reeling me in.

I set out to India with more than $30,000 worth of equipment. Of course, the customs officer in the Bombay airport, sensing a big financial bonanza, wanted to charge import duty despite my telling him it was all charitable donations. I started praying for Swami's help. Just then the supervisor arrived. The second he heard it was for Swami's hospital, he ordered his men not only to help pack the sutures in a suitcase, but to help transport everything to the domestic terminal for the trip to Madras. Swami is always testing one's faith, but He will always come to the rescue at the bleakest moment.

I met my wife and children and went for morning darshan in Whitefield, near Bangalore. The first thing that is most striking is the difference in atmosphere as one crosses the gates into Brindavan. What a serene, safe, and clean atmosphere! Being a little late, we sat way back in the sun, but I could still see Swami as He gave darshan and then sat for bhajans. What a privilege it was singing directly to God, not to a picture or an idol. We came back for afternoon darshan, and the next day I set off on my mission to visit the Sri Sathya Sai Institute of Higher Medical Sciences (SSSIHMS).

The trip to Puttaparthi from Bangalore is long, dusty, and dangerous. Only Swami's grace can get you there in one piece. I will never forget the first time I saw the hospital. In a vast expanse of desert, you go up a hill, and on the other side is an absolutely breathtaking view. The hospital really looks like a temple. The pastel colors, the symmetry, and the beauty give it a surreal appearance. We passed through the gates, and I have never received such a heartwarming welcome. It looked like everybody knew me. They made me immediately feel like part of the Sai family. I met most of the hospital staff, which was quite small, as cardiology and cardiac surgery were the only divisions open. The head of the blood bank was overflowing with love and asked me to give a talk on any subject of my choice. I just happened to have with me a talk on heart transplantation, with slides I had prepared, because my father-in-law had set up a meeting with the Rotary Club in his city. The slides had accidentally been included with the equipment I took to Puttaparthi. After the talk and a truly uplifting visit to SSSIHMS, I returned to Bangalore on an emotional high. The staff was inspiring, compassionate, and full of Swami stories. It was as if I had spent all that time with Swami Himself. The next morning, we went early for darshan, and I could see Swami up close. He looked at me with a sweet smile, and I felt shock waves going through me. I was stunned. There was so much energy and love. Swami took our letters, and we returned home basking in His blessings.

We increased our participation in service projects and regularly attended bhajans. Then, about three months later, I received a letter that profoundly changed my life. It was an invitation to speak at the Second International Symposium on Cardiovascular Medicine at Puttaparthi. Apparently my previous talk on heart transplantation had made an impression, and they wanted me to talk on that subject again. What an incredible honor bestowed upon me by Swami! I was a little intimidated, as there were many leading and eminent doctors invited to speak. Why a young, unaccomplished surgeon such as myself? That is just one of Swami's many leelas. Eventually, the day came for me to leave. It was a miserable day with snow and ice. Other travelers from around where I lived could only make the journey several days later. With Swami's grace, not only did I get to the airport in an ice storm, but also every connection was perfect. It was all His grace.

I had the privilege of being able to sit on the veranda during morning darshan. I could see Swami up close and feel His incredible love. A cardiologist and myself struck up a friendship and discussed how we became part of Swami's "team." After selecting people for interviews, Swami came to us and told us to leave and have breakfast. Realizing that the conference did not start for another hour, we decided to stay seated for another opportunity to see Swami. Trading breakfast to be in Swami's presence seemed like a great idea. Eventually we went to eat and arrived at the conference hall 15 minutes before the start of the proceedings. Strangely, none of the other doctors were present. We sat down, and then they all arrived together with Swami. They had all eaten early and then come to the lecture hall with Swami. He had given them a group interview and personal messages. It was then that I realized why Swami had wanted us to leave and eat breakfast. Swami knows so many things that are beyond our comprehension. We think on a worldly scale; He knows on a cosmic scale. That was the last time I ever disobeyed Swami.

There were about 30 doctors giving talks at the conference. Swami gave a discourse on ways to prevent heart disease. All illnesses, Swami said, can be attributed to one of three reasons: hurry, worry, and curry. Swami proceeded to praise the work of doctors, then made some piercing remarks. He said that doctors have been given respect for studying hard and obtaining degrees. But is it deserved? Do they practice with compassion and understanding? Talking to patients can be the best cure. Making a good living is acceptable, but do charity work as well. Donate a percentage of your time to the needy. Those dictums of Swami's were like an arrow piercing my heart. Since that time, I have become much less materialistic. With His grace, we lead a very comfortable life, but we do not fixate on money. What a personal transformation! Furthermore, since that time, I have treated all patients, regardless of their ability to pay. Some of my toughest and longest cases have been ones done gratis. All patients are treated with the best care, using the best possible techniques. I show the same compassion to every single patient. Swami has given me the strength just to concentrate on the best possible job I can do for each patient. He has given me a rare gift: the ability to be a surgeon and help patients. I just want to use this gift to serve mankind. That is not to say that I totally disregard the business of medicine. That is not realistic. We always have to negotiate the best possible deals with insurance companies, but the driving force is not money but how to best serve each patient.

During the conference, Swami played the role of host to perfection. Every night there was a performance by the students. The food was delicious, especially because Swami talked to us as we were served. Swami is very compassionate but can also be strict and demanding. For instance, when not in Puttaparthi, doctors rarely sit through an entire medical meeting. Most doctors usually attend what interests them and then disappear to relax or sightsee. A group of us left the afternoon sessions and went to darshan. Swami immediately wanted to know why we were there and not attending the meeting. I attended every subsequent session. That is the only conference I have been to where attendance throughout the day was close to 100 percent. I learned so much in fields in which I had no prior interest. Although I was invited to discuss my area of expertise, I felt I learned much more than when I was teaching. This involved learning about the morality and spirituality of medicine, as well as about the science of medicine. I had a very interesting experience during one of the nightly plays. I had brought my camera, which was a Canon EOS with an automatic focus zoom lens. Swami arrived and, being less than 10 feet away, I had a great opportunity for a picture. He looked toward me and smiled. What a great shot! But my camera would not focus. The lens kept going to the infinity setting. Swami kept looking and laughing. My desperate attempts at focusing were thwarted by a runaway camera. Just then Swami said, laughingly, *Camera can't focus.* He laughed and turned away. At that moment my usually reliable camera snapped back into focus. Swami was playing with me, showing that His power is infinite and everything is His will.

The meeting ended, and I had to stay an extra day to catch my flight back to the United States. In the morning, Swami granted me an interview. I had not expected this, although I had previously written down a list of questions in case I was granted this privilege. I went to the interview room with several others whom I do not remember, and with Dr. Donald Ross, probably one of the greatest surgeons in the world. Imagine me, an upstart, sitting next to this luminary. Only Swami can pull these diverse groups of people together. I had practiced all my questions and was "ready for Swami." Of course, the second I went inside, I completely melted. I was totally overwhelmed. I sat down across from Swami, and He started talking about very practical things such as money, family, and work. By this time I had completely forgotten about my "wish list," but Swami went right down the list, item by item. It was as if He were reading what I had written. He truly knows everything. Two items come to mind about that interview. Swami made a repeated point about money. He stressed that money will come and go. It is necessary, but not something to worry about. He told us not to worry about the future but, rather, to enjoy the present. He also discussed patients. I work very hard on my patients and do technically perfect operations, yet some of them die. Swami said that He knows I try very hard, but that life and death are not in my hands, but in His. It is His responsibility, as well as the patient's karma. I just need to do my best; the rest is up to Him. He took all of that responsibility out of my hands. Of course, I have to be responsible, careful, and meticulous. Swami supplies the divine energy force that lets a lot of patients who come to me, after being denied surgery by others, survive. Swami went on to say that, whatever the patient's karma, it cannot be changed, and that death may actually be the most humane thing for that particular patient.

Since that interview, I have become much more comfortable discussing God's work with my patients. Many of them are desperately ill and come to our institution because their cases are hopeless. I tell the patients that, although I will do my best, there is certainly a chance they may die, and that God is the one who determines that. I am just a humble instrument of God's action. I try to steer their hopes away from me and have them focus on God. Remarkably, the patients who truly believe in God and say they will completely leave it "in the hands of God" have recovered remarkably well. This is the power of faith and prayer. For example, I had a patient who had been suffering with heart failure for six months.

Having been denied surgery elsewhere, he came to us for a fourth opinion. We operated on him, and he did remarkably well until the fifth day, when he suddenly died. I was devastated, but his wife was calm. She said that her husband had suffered for a long time. His quality of life was dismal. All he wanted was a chance, and he received that. Death, she said, was better than his suffering in life. She thanked me for giving him a chance and letting him finally find peace.

At the end of the interview, Swami gave me some vibhuti, and I left for Bangalore. I had put some very precious things in a bag: Swami's vibhuti, other mementos from the conference, and some pictures presented to me by a doctor who, in turn, had received them from Swami. I checked into the hotel in Bangalore and went to the airport at night for a flight to Bombay. To my horror, I had misplaced the bag. I probably left it in the taxi from Puttaparthi. There was no way to retrieve it. I told my contact about this at the Bangalore airport about 30 minutes before departure. However, no one even knew which taxi I had traveled in from Puttaparthi. I felt I had lost the most precious things in life. I got on the plane, and the doors closed. Then there was a delay. I was getting a little anxious, as I had a connection to make. Just then, the doors reopened, and airline officials asked if I was on board. I thought I must be in a lot of trouble. A person came to me, dropped off the bag with all of my precious belongings, and left. I did not know him, nor did any of my Bangalore contacts with whom I later spoke. This was another one of Swami's miracles!

When I arrived in Philadelphia, my wife, Sheela, was very anxious. She told me that one of our investments had gone sour and the sponsor had swindled our money. She then waited for me to explode. I remembered Swami had specifically made a point of discussing money. To Sheela's astonishment, I took the large loss in stride, which was completely contrary to my previous behavior. Swami continually leads us down the righteous path; we just have to follow.

During the summer, a Dr. Venugopal came to Temple University to be trained in heart transplantation. He had planned to stay a week, and I had warned him that transplantation is very erratic. Sometimes one does not occur for two to three weeks or more. Swami had blessed his trip and told him when to go. Miraculously, when Dr. Venugopal arrived at his hotel in Philadelphia, we had started a transplant. The pace stayed that way for a total of four or five days. One could not have asked for a better period for training. During his visit, I asked him about the possibility of my working in Puttaparthi. Dr. Venugopal had set up the program at the SSSIHMS, and his team did all the surgery in the early years. What a spectacular group of people! They all went during their vacations and did innumerable operations. Dr. Venugopal's vision and pursuit of perfection are what made the heart surgery section what it is today.

I was granted permission to work at the SSSIHMS and decided to go in the beginning of 1995. After the usual drama going through customs, I arrived in Puttaparthi in February, during the Shivarathri celebrations. At that time, the fulltime staff at the hospital was relatively inexperienced. Surgeons would come with entire teams (surgeons, assistants, anesthesiologists, nurses), operate on a lot of patients, and leave. Patients were getting great care, but after a team left, there was a lull in the number of surgeries being performed. I was one of the few surgeons who came on my own. Through Swami's grace, the whole Puttaparthi team rallied together, and we got a lot accomplished. In the beginning, I did most of the cases then, slowly, I started teaching the staff surgeons. We did more than 20 cases, a combination of valve replacements and coronary bypass surgeries, in a little more than a week.

The hospital truly is a unique place on earth. Built in less than one year, it is a testament to Swami's will and the human spirit. It appears more like a temple than a hospital. What is really impressive is the staff. Many of them have no experience or official schooling in the duties they perform. For instance, the perfusionists, the specialists who operate the heart/lung machine, are graduates of Swami's business school. Swami picked them out and directed them to the All-India Institute of Medical Sciences in New Delhi for training under Dr. Venugopal's team. They are now some of the best perfusionists that one could ever work with. They have also been very innovative in making the heart/lung machine both cost efficient and better for patient care. The same is true of the nurses and support personnel. They have been placed there by Swami to do this work. Being close to Him and participating in His mission are adequate rewards for them. Out of compassion and without regard to money, the surgeons have also made a big sacrifice. They could have made exponentially more money working anywhere else in the country. But where else would they have access to great equipment, treat patients with a vast variety of illnesses and have God's daily blessing? Over the years, they have gained a lot of experience and developed into top-notch surgeons. Dedication and compassion make this institute truly unique. Patients are considered as people, not as a source of revenue.

People often ask me how Swami's hospital compares to other hospitals. It not only has technology, but it also has compassion and love. The question should be reversed. How could any other hospital ever compare to SSSIHMS? However, not everything is perfect. There are so many people requiring care that the waiting list approaches 50,000 patients. In essence, the patients pay by waiting. Only a small percentage of patients can actually have treatment. Sometimes, it is not even the wait. One time a surgeon brought pacemakers, and I brought homograft valves. Each item cost more than $10,000. Of the 30 or so telegrams that were sent to patients to get them admitted during our visit, only five or so actually arrived. A few had died, but most did not have the $3 bus fare to come to Puttaparthi. What a sad situation! I asked the staff about this. Swami has told them to do the best they can. The waiting list will never go away. Swami built the hospital as an example to which everyone should aspire. It is a model of what should be built around the world. Swami wants others to follow His lead and build similar institutions in every corner of the globe.

Daily, we operated late into the night. We slowed down during the Shivarathri celebrations. That actually made me a little upset, because I wanted to demonstrate how many cases we could do. I should have realized that Swami was just giving us a break to relax, but only in retrospect could I appreciate His grace. Swami, of course, is very protective of the hospital and the patients. He often asks how many cases were performed and how the patients are doing. If any of the operating room staff goes to evening darshan, Swami immediately inquires as to the reason. He expects a full day's work and does not want staff to finish early, even if it is to attend darshan.

Toward the end of my visit, I was hit with the interview virus. Everyone was concerned that I had not yet been called. Other surgeons had been given multiple interviews; why had I not? This only heightened my anxieties. An interview would be nice and would be the icing on the cake, but I had come to serve and operate. Having the ability to help people was the ultimate reward.

Sitting down for Swami's darshan is probably the most spiritually therapeutic medicine in the world. I start to think of all the ways I should improve: show more compassion, eliminate jealousy, be more cheerful, feel less anger. The list goes on. Even amongst the crowd, I felt solitude; it is just you, Swami, and all your inner feelings. I realized that Swami is actually more therapeutic if He ignores you. That makes you look within and see if there are things to do to get back in His good graces. I was reading a book during morning darshan, and two passages were especially important. The author was describing the "monkey mind." In one story, a monkey puts his hands in a jar and grabs some nuts. His hand cannot come out of the jar. All he needs to do is release the nuts, but he cannot let go. It is symbolic of man's inability to let go of desires in order to attain freedom and peace. Just as I finished the passage, I looked up, and what was there, sitting on the wall, but a monkey. I have tried ever since to tame my monkey mind. That is clearly a job that still requires a lot of work.

The next important passage in the book was about a devotee's experience with Swami. In one interview, he received a diamond ring. I found myself thinking about how special that must have been. Meanwhile, Swami gave darshan and then went into the interview room with a group of devotees. Just before closing the door, He came back out and mischievously grinned at me and motioned for me to join them. My parents came as well. Once inside, Swami had a big laugh making fun of my doubts and anxieties, and told me my mind had a lot of confusion. He said, *Just remember, Swami will give.* Interviews or dialogues with Swami are usually not direct advice. They tend to be phrases that can be interpreted in many ways. We have to look within ourselves and be guided by Swami's to find the right meaning. It dawned on me later that Swami does give, except it is not always what or when we expect. The adage, "Be careful what you wish, for it may come true," is certainly appropriate. For instance, there have been many times in the operating room when I have prayed to Swami to make a patient's heart pump better, let them survive and be able to leave the operating room. Some of those patients have gone on to have perfect hearts, but then to suffer from strokes, infections, pneumonia, or kidney and liver failure. Some have truly suffered for a long time before finally dying. I have learned that one needs to surrender completely to Swami. Let Him decide what is right at any given time. He knows all of eternity. We see only the past and present, truly a microcosm. Surrender to Him and life becomes very peaceful. Our mission is to be compassionate and loving and to serve mankind. When intentions are pure, Swami fills in everything else.

Swami went around and talked to several devotees during the initial group interview. He materialized vibhuti, which is a fascinating experience. He waves His hand, palm down, in a circular motion and then turns His palm up and distributes vibhuti with His fingers. Normally, vibhuti is a gray, very light powder, and will scatter if poured. Swami's vibhuti is pure white and falls into your hand onto a concentrated spot without a particle scattering. Furthermore, it tastes different to each individual. Some say it is sweet, some say it is milky, and some say it is tart.

After a while, Swami looked at me and said, *Doctor.* He was smiling, loving, and letting me know He knows everything on my mind. He asked me what I wanted. I was too stunned to answer. With a wave of His hand, He materialized a ring. It was a diamond ring, which is what I had thought of while reading the book before darshan. He put it on my right hand and said, *Perfect fit.* Swami always makes the rings fit perfectly. It was a beautiful, solitary stone ring. Since I operate daily and am afraid of losing it, I have worn it as a necklace ever since that magical day. When Swami put it on my hand, He said the word "diamond." It was only later that I realized that "diamond" actually is symbolic for "die mind;" and as Swami has said, if one lets his mind die, one will attain peace and freedom.

We were then called in for a private interview. This time it was much more personal. Swami made us sit close to Him. He took my right hand, rested it on His lap and massaged my fingers, and then held both my hands tight. He playfully slapped my back, rubbed my chest, and blessed me. He spoke to my mother and asked about her trip to Thirupathi. She said that, when she saw the deity there, she could see only Swami's figure. He confirmed that He was there. Whatever temple you visit, He is there. Going to Puttaparthi and seeing Swami is the ultimate pilgrimage. In a temple, you pray to a deity; at Prasanthi Nilayam, you see the living God Himself. My parents then asked for one of Swami's robes, and He said, *I will give.* As I wrote before, Swami always gives, we just do not know when or where. This time, we were destined to wait.

We went back to the United States with recharged spirits. On the plane home, I had the opportunity to think about several Sai medical miracles that I have personally encountered. We had a patient at Temple University who had a massive heart attack, became very unstable, and was rushed to surgery. He needed several important blood vessels bypassed but, when his chest was opened, we found that the heart attack had been so big that all the usual landmarks we use to find the vessels were completely obliterated. I searched for more than 20 minutes without finding any vessels. Everyone in the operating room was getting nervous for, if those vessels could not be found and bypassed, the patient would surely die. I was dissecting on the back of the heart to find the vessels, frustration and anxiety mounting. Just then, I heard the words, "Sai Ram." No one else in the room was a Baba devotee, so those words startled me. In addition, I felt a sharp pinch in the middle of my chest just where I wear Swami's materialized ring as a necklace. My hand moved involuntarily, and I made a cut in the patient's heart. Right there, in an area where we never would have found it, was the main artery. Two others were found quickly, and the patient did very well. Everyone in the operating room wanted to know how I had done that. I told them it was luck, but that it was helpful to have God on our side. Clearly, I was acting as an instrument of the Lord. Ever since then, I have, on occasion, felt a pinch on my chest in the exact spot where the ring is touching me. Of course, this makes me instantly think of Swami.

In 1998, I was a participant in another Sai medical miracle. Dr. Girishankar had a history of problems with one of his heart valves. In 1993, physicians insisted that he should have surgery, and he went to Puttaparthi to seek Swami's permission. Swami told him to postpone surgery and "lose weight." Imaging of the heart after the visit to Puttaparthi revealed significant improvement. Surgery was postponed, and he felt good. Five years later, Mrs. Girishankar was anxious about her husband's worsening condition. She mentioned her concern to a Sai friend who recommended contacting me. A few months later, the Girishankars made an appointment and came to my office. We talked more about Swami than about Mr. Girishankar's medical condition. His valve was bad, and the heart was starting to deteriorate. This was the best time for surgery. They wanted Swami's permission, and they received it in the form of a dream in which Swami blessed the surgery. We did an angiogram before surgery and, to everyone's surprise, it showed that there were blocked arteries. If he had undergone surgery five years earlier, he would have needed another operation by this time. Despite what conventional medical wisdom had dictated, Swami had saved him from having an extra operation. They wanted the surgery to be on a Thursday, and we were able to accommodate them. Mr. Girishankar was put to sleep by the anesthesiologist. He and his wife had asked me to put vibhuti on his forehead and tongue. Since there were about ten people in the room, I braced myself for a barrage of questions and ridicule. I just prayed to Swami, took the vibhuti, and placed some on his forehead and the tip of his tongue. Everyone was looking at me, but not one person said a word. It was as if they did not see me do it. As I scrubbed for the surgery, I prayed to Swami to guide me through the operation. These are difficult operations not only because of the multiple procedures on the heart, but also because of the emotional attachment to a Sai devotee. I asked Swami to give me a sign that He was there with me in the operating room. Just then, our chief of neurosurgery walked in. We had not spoken for about four months. It seems that he had a visitor awhile back who had given him a picture of Swami. He had meant to give it to me but had never found the time. Despite all these months, he happened to remember it that particular day. When he gave me the picture, I noticed it had a saying on it that read, "May divine grace and blessings be ever with you in all your noble deeds." Swami always answers your prayers; one only needs to be alert to get the message. The surgery went beautifully. Swami was there guiding everyone in the operating room. The patient made a remarkable recovery and has done perfectly since.

Another story involves Arunan Sivalingum, an eminent retinal specialist. At the young age of 37, Arunan was considered one of the foremost ophthalmologists in the world. He was health conscious, despite leading a very busy and stressful life. He experienced some nausea and vomiting and went to the emergency room at his institution. The most likely diagnosis was an ulcer, so he was being prepared to receive a gastroscopy. As a part of the routine, he also had an EKG, which showed a massive heart attack. He was rushed to the cardiology suite, and an angiogram revealed massive coronary artery disease. He became unstable and was rushed to the operating room. The surgeons performed bypass surgery but were unsuccessful in recovering the heart. They placed him on a temporary heart-assist device and debated what to do with this dying patient. This is where Sai incidents take over. It so happened that one of the doctors in charge of the intensive care unit had just attended our conferences on transplantation and end-stage heart disease. She immediately encouraged the surgeons to refer him to us at Temple. In addition, Arunan's wife was best friends with the wife of our medical director of transplantation. Arunan was transferred early in the morning and went directly to our operating room. He was unconscious, was on a ventilator, had his chest open, was bleeding, and had poor blood flow. The mortality rate of such a patient is about 80 percent. I took one look at him and my heart sank. Here was an important member of society, a young, energetic husband and a father of four, including a newborn. Only a miracle could save him. Just then, the nurses pulled back the sheets in preparation for surgery. There was a picture of Swami. Arunan's mother, a long time devotee, had taped a picture of our Swami to his upper arm. My nurses were surprised. They exclaimed, "Hey, that's the dude in the picture at your house Val." I started thinking that maybe now we had a chance. We started the surgery and proceeded to stop the bleeding, take out the temporary device, and implant a more permanent artificial heart. The idea was to get him better and wait until a heart transplant could be done. The surgery was tricky, and we barely got him through. He was transferred to the intensive care unit in grave condition. The slightest complication would mean death. He remained unstable.

I had to go to a very important meeting in San Francisco that I had postponed attending many times. I left him in my partner's capable hands and boarded the cross-country flight. Arunan continued to bleed, but his blood flows were acceptable. I kept in constant contact by sky phone. Then, his flow started to go down. He was starting to die. Opening his chest again would surely have killed him. I gave a bunch of orders, but things were looking bleak. At that time, my plane began its descent into San Francisco, and the sky phones were shut off. The only option was to pray. I told Swami that Arunan was completely in His hands. There was nothing we could do. That was around 6:00 p.m. on the West Coast. I went to the hotel room fully expecting disaster. I called the hospital in Philadelphia and spoke to the resident, who was giddy with happiness. At exactly 9:00 p.m., 6:00 p.m. on the West Coast, and also Swami's special number, a miracle had happened. Arunan stopped bleeding, and his blood flows improved dramatically. By the next day, he was off the critical list and did spectacularly well with the device. He ended up going home and even operated on patients while on the device. It was truly a miracle.

That was only the beginning. He was on the device without any complications, which is rare, for more than nine months. With Swami's guidance, I was contemplating a career move to Chicago. But I felt a personal responsibility to have Arunan's transplant done before I left Philadelphia. During a Sunday bhajan, I prayed hard to Swami. I did not want to leave without finishing what we had started on Arunan. During meditation, my beeper went off. A heart was available, but there were seven people ahead of Arunan. I told the coordinator to send blood for matches on everyone. The coordinator asked twice about sending blood on Arunan because he was so far down on the list. I insisted. Through divine grace, every one of the patients above him tested poorly. Swami had designated this heart for Arunan. We proceeded with the transplant. I placed vibhuti on

Arunan and, again, there were more than 15 people in the room watching, but no one actually saw me do it. The transplant was truly divine. It went without a hitch. I could feel Swami taking over the operation. There was no other way for it to go so perfectly. The new heart jumped back to life. Everyone in the room was absolutely amazed; this was the best heart anyone had seen. Arunan has done great since then and, with Swami overlooking things, he will continue to do so. He has become a strong devotee and has sent his curriculum vitae to Swami to ask for permission to work at the hospital in Puttaparthi. I am sure that Swami will get him there one day. Swami has always said He will open His hands, and the best doctors will come. They just come at different times and by different paths.

My next experience was during the third cardiovascular symposium. The number of physicians who had been invited to attend the conference had grown exponentially. It was a great meeting, and I was able to talk to many experts in the field. One day during lunch, Swami came into the cafeteria. Everyone stood up, and Swami motioned for all to sit. People sat down momentarily, but then stood up again. Swami just turned around and left. The next day, He came again and motioned for us to sit. Not one person got up. We had all learned our lesson. We always need to follow Swami's direction.

The last day of the meeting, Swami came to the cafeteria and started distributing pictures that were taken of the doctors with Him. He gave me, along with two other surgeons, the stack of pictures for us to distribute. To my disappointment, I could not find a picture of myself with Swami. I just accepted this and did not give it a second thought. However, during afternoon darshan, Swami came close to me and stopped. He motioned to one of the students, who then ran to Swami's residence and came back with some pictures. Swami handed them to me. On top was a beautiful snapshot of Swami presenting me with a trophy that He personally gives to each participant of the symposium. I was so elated and felt really special. But that feeling was to be abolished very quickly. Swami has a way of eliminating the ego and the harmful feelings it creates.

As it was the end of the conference, we were asked to vacate our flat in the North block. Despite suggestions that we move to a similar accommodation in Prasanthi Nilayam, I had asked to stay at the guesthouse at the hospital. That 5 km trip, through a comedy of errors, took four hours. The guesthouse had obviously not been used recently; it was dirty, smelly, and full of cockroaches. We did not settle in until after midnight. The next day, during morning darshan, Swami smiled at me slightly and asked if we were finally settled in. He knew about the trials of the night before. He just keeps everyone on their toes. The only thing predictable about Swami is His unpredictability. With Swami, nobody is special. We are all equal. It is just that we have different karma and roles that we are destined to play in this world, all as part of Swami's leela.

I helped with several surgeries that day. The next day was the final morning at Puttaparthi, and Swami, as usual, waited until the last possible minute to call us for an interview. This time it was with my wife, children, and parents in a most personal interview. We all sat in front of Swami. He blessed us all. He said He was always with us. My parents asked again for a robe, and Swami said, *I will give.* After the personal interview was finished, everyone sat together as a group. Swami asked me what I wanted. I was speechless. He then materialized a beautiful bracelet that He put on my right hand. I never used to wear jewelry, no matter how valuable or beautiful. Now, with Swami's grace, I am wearing all of His divine gifts. The bracelet is always with me, either on my wrist or, when I operate, in my pocket. Taking it off and on always reminds me to pray to Swami before every surgery.

Swami then went to the inside room and came back with two robes. My father had asked for them, and he was most anxious to get one. Swami went directly to him, then turned at the last moment and gave the robes to my wife and my mother. My father was so disappointed. Swami then materialized vibhuti for the ladies, and the interview was over. Just then, Swami went to His inner room and, laughing, came back with a robe for Dad. Playfully, He said that my father had looked so sad. Our compassionate Swami!

Fifteen months later, I returned to India with my assistant and operated for ten days. We performed and assisted on many cases. The last case was the most memorable. Dr. Parsed, the chief cardiologist, presented a case to us saying that it was a difficult one. I told him it was easy and actually said it would be done in two hours. We had all types of problems during this case, and we struggled to get the patient off the operating room table. He eventually did well but, after that case, I stopped being so cocky and arrogant. Anything can happen at any time. Swami's will is in control, not we mortal beings. We can never assume anything, only that Swami will always be with us.

Again, Swami graced us with an interview at the absolute last moment. When He asked me what I wanted, I said, "Your blessings," and He told me that I always had them. He asked again, and I said, "Your grace," and He gave me the same answer. Finally, I said, "Whatever you desire Swami." He materialized a silver ring with an Om sign. He asked what silver meant. *Purity,* He replied. He then took back the ring, blew on it and it became gold, with His picture on it. He put it on my finger; again, a perfect fit. During our personal interview, Swami had asked where my diamond ring was. I told Him that I wore it as a necklace. He then took off the ring that He had just materialized, blew on it, and it disappeared. I guess if you don't use it, you lose it. Swami then asked about my work. "Fine," I said. He responded, *No good, too much jealousy.* That was the first time Swami had said that there was a problem with work. Externally, everything was perfect. We had built a new house, I was director of the largest transplant program in the United States, and my career, with Swami's grace, was blossoming. But Swami knew, and He clearly predicted the future. He then materialized a nine gem (Navaratna) ring for me, which I wear along with the other ring, on a necklace.

After the interview, we went to a friend's house. His wife commented on my ring and said it must be the latest model. Swami had materialized a similar ring for her, but one of the stones had fallen out. My friend later told me that, after our departure, his wife wanted him to ask Swami to fix the ring. He told his wife to ask for herself. That evening, during darshan, Swami asked them to stay and come for an interview the next morning. During the interview, the first thing Swami asked about was the ring. He fixed it right there and gave it back. Swami is omnipresent. Whether it is our thoughts or conversations, He knows. If you consider that, then all thoughts, actions, and words will become pure.

As predicted, the next year did bring a lot of changes at work. There was instability in our department, as our chief stopped looking out for the best interests of our program. I was invited to speak at the Indian Association of Thoracic Surgery at Jaipur. I wrote a letter asking for Swami's permission to work at SSSIHMS at the end of February. Usually, a reply arrives in about a month. In January, I became nervous. I did not want to go without Swami's permission. Just then, I received word that the IATS conference was delayed, due to an emergency election, until the end of March. When I asked again for permission, a positive reply was sent within a week. Swami knows every single detail. I was destined to go in late March, and that is when I went. Just before I was to leave for India, I received a call from the University of Chicago asking me if I would be interested in interviewing for the position of Chief of Cardiothoracic Surgery. I wanted to postpone speaking to them until after the trip to India, but they insisted, so I went for a day. Certainly, being asked to be the department chief at a very young age, in such a prestigious institution, could only be influenced by Swami's hand. I was happy to be asked, but Temple University countered with a similar offer, and it was going to be much easier to stay where I was. When I arrived in India, Swami was in Whitefield, and I saw Him on Sunday before going off to Puttaparthi. Although it was not the same without morning darshan, work started earlier, and we got a lot of cases done. My role had really changed over the years. I was now mainly an educator and teacher, not the primary surgeon. Because I was immersed in work, the week flew by.

On the day I was to leave, I fully anticipated another of Swami's usual leelas, figuring He would postpone the interview until the last possible minute. Of course, He was as unpredictable as always. The second I passed through the gates of Brindavan, several devotees came directly to me and said Swami wanted to see me for an interview in the morning. Swami started with the usual, *How are you, doctor?* He then went ahead and solved one of my main dilemmas. When we perform bypass surgery, it is conventional practice to use veins as grafts for the procedure. I like to use arteries instead, as they are naturally meant to handle high pressure. Veins are obtained from the legs; they are long, and easy to work with. Arteries are obtained from the arm (radial), chest wall (internal thoracic), or the stomach (gastroepiploic); they are much shorter and less forgiving in terms of length. Why not maintain the artery in its natural state instead of transforming a low-pressure vessel, such as a vein, into an artery? It is much more technically demanding and tricky to do this, so only about 5 percent of cardiac surgeons do this type of operation routinely. In my practice, and at SSIHMS, we had implemented a system of using arterial grafts as much as possible. However, there is no way to prove if this is better, and we won't know for at least five to ten years. I've always wondered whether the extra effort was worth it but, despite the lack of conclusive medical data, I believed in my heart that it was. In the interview, Swami first spoke to a businessman and told him to lose weight, otherwise he would require bypass surgery. Then Swami answered my dilemma by describing how I do not use veins, that I use arteries, which is a better and more advanced technique. I no longer need scientific proof. Swami validated all of the extra work involved in using arterial grafts.

He then asked me what I wanted, and materialized another bracelet, much larger than the first. While putting it on, He taught me a lesson. The previous day, I had become impatient and taken over in a case in order to speed up the stitching of some of the bypasses. At times, I tend to be impatient with instructing people. When Swami was putting the bracelet on me and fumbling with the latch, I was going to offer my help in putting it on. Then it struck me that Swami was sending me a message: be patient with others. Since then, I have really tried to change my ways.

While Swami had personal interviews with other devotees, I was wondering what to do with two bracelets. Swami finally invited us into the inner room. This time, I was full of questions. I started asking Him about Chicago and, before I could finish, He took my hand in His, told me He knew about the move, that He had arranged it, and that I must go. It was a direct command from the divine. Then, before I could ask, He told me to take off the smaller bracelet and keep it in front of His picture at home. He said the newer bracelet was the latest design, was permanent, and the most powerful. As you can imagine, the rest of the interview was a blur.

We, indeed, moved from Philadelphia to Chicago. It would never have happened without Swami being so forceful. Every time I thought of all the things we were giving up in Philadelphia, Swami's words came to mind. From a practical point of view, the move did not make sense. The program was more established at Temple University; I made more money there, we had an incomparable house; and I had the respect of the community. But faith in Swami and His forceful words made the move possible. At one point, I was really having doubts, and I wrote a letter to Swami from my office. I asked for a sign that this move really was what He meant. Just then, my secretary knocked and said a Dr. Mulder was calling. I told her to take a message, but Dr. Mulder was persistent. I took the call, and he said he was an alumnus of the surgery department of the University of Chicago. He gave me a ten-minute discourse on why I should move. I later found out that no one at the University of Chicago knew of a Dr. Mulder. It was Swami Himself giving the sign I had wanted. He always answers our prayers, just in different ways than one would expect.

This is just a small sampling of my experiences with Bhagavan Baba. Since I have witnessed and participated in Swami's miracles, my entire attitude toward life has changed. I have been taught humility, compassion, and to serve mankind. Swami sets high standards, and I do not know if I can ever reach them. But, with His guidance, I have been directed onto the right path. I have a long way to go, but my Lord and guru, Sai Baba, will surely get me there.

Practicing Medicine With Sai
Charles Bollmann, M.D.

It was January 1978, and I had just returned from my first trip to India to see Sai Baba. It had been the greatest experience of my life. Things were going well. I had a thriving practice in obstetrics and gynecology in Phoenix, Arizona, and my wife and I had just celebrated the birth of a daughter. I did not expect the turn of events that occurred with a patient who became the ultimate challenge.

Terry's first pregnancy had progressed normally until about six weeks before her due date. As her obstetrician, I was surprised to get a call from the hospital that she was in labor. The delivery was uneventful, and the baby, while premature, was doing well. On returning to my office, the post-partum nurse called and informed me Terry's blood pressure was markedly elevated. While making rounds the next morning, I realized Terry's laboratory findings were extremely abnormal. In essence, all of the liver-function tests were elevated. For a healthy female of 26 years, this was extremely unusual.

Consultation with an internal medicine physician was obtained but, before the diagnosis could be determined, Terry developed a postpartum hemorrhage. This required returning her to the operating room where a D & C was performed. By this time, additional laboratory studies were returned revealing almost no platelets present. The diagnosis of Disseminated Intravascular Coagulation (DIC - a disease that prevents blood from clotting) was made, and a hematology consultation was obtained. Platelets and whole blood were transfused. The diagnosis of a rare disorder, acute yellow atrophy of the liver in pregnancy, was made. This is a condition in which the liver is almost completely replaced by fat cells and is unable to function. The cause is unknown, and the condition is extremely rare.

The next morning, because of the lack of clotting factors, Terry developed an extremely large hematoma, a collection of blood, into the episiotomy site. She again required transfusions and was taken back to the operating room where the hematoma was evacuated. As her condition progressively deteriorated, I reviewed the sparse medical literature about the condition. I was able to find only five articles in the entire medical literature. By the fourth article, I realized that there was no mention of prognosis, or the outcome of the condition, in any of the articles. Apparently, this was because everyone died - the disease was fatal. Since no one can live without a liver, Terry's condition rapidly deteriorated. Another postpartum hemorrhage developed, and I was required to perform a hysterectomy to control the bleeding.

Despite my efforts and those of 10 other specialists in various fields, we continued to lose ground. Terry developed a hemorrhage from the stomach and gastrointestinal (GI) tract, renal failure, and a stress ulcer. She went into congestive heart failure and, finally, coma. During this time, she received 155 units of platelets, 55 units of packed cells (blood transfusion), five units of fresh whole blood, and multiple units of fresh frozen plasma. During all this she remained in a coma. I asked Sai Baba to help her and me to get through this, and I gave her vibhuti. I began to wonder if her purpose in life was to provide me with a crash course in every medical emergency known to man.

After four weeks, Terry's case was taking up all my time; my practice was suffering, and I was neglecting my wife and new baby. Finally, I was able to attend a medical meeting in Scottsdale, the town adjacent to Phoenix. I had been at the meeting for only an hour when the intensive-care nurse paged me. Terry had suffered a cardiac arrest. Speeding back to the hospital in Phoenix, I arrived to find Terry resuscitated and alive but still comatose.

I asked Swami to help me. I drew the curtain around the bed and began to talk to the comatose Terry. I explained that the situation could not continue as it was, that it was interfering with my life, my other patients, and my newborn child. I explained that she had a lot to live for, with her husband and their new baby, but I insisted she make a decision one way or the other. Her options were to die or to recover, but she needed to make a decision so that I could get on with my life. I could not continue to dedicate all my time to her and neglect my other patients and my own family.

I returned to my office to see patients. Within an hour, the intensive-care nurse called and excitedly told me that Terry had awakened from the coma. Two days later, she left the intensive-care unit and, within one week, she returned home with her baby. Six weeks later, her liver function was entirely normal. I know that the results would have been different had Swami not had His hand in the matter. Certainly, none of the other specialists or I did anything magical to save Terry. This was my first assurance that Swami would always be there to guide me in caring for my patients, and this has lasted throughout my medical career.

Raised a Catholic, I entered the seminary to become a priest at an early age. After two years, I realized it was not for me. I then spent my junior and senior years at a Catholic high school in New Jersey, attended Villanova University in Pennsylvania, and then attended the University of Medicine, in New Jersey, for my medical degree. Residency training and a busy medical practice kept me busy for several years, but I was always on the "spiritual path." I simply did not have time to pursue it; there was so much to learn.

Finally, I felt I was enough of an expert in medicine to get back to what I was really interested in - metaphysics. I started studying all types of spiritual knowledge and paths, from Scientology to est. I read *Autobiography of a Yogi* by Paramahamsa Yogananda, books by Ram Dass and Carlos Castaneda, as well as others by Ramakrishna and Ramana Maharshi. I knew I had to go to India but did not know where to go. While visiting a bookstore in Del Mar, California, I found a small section of metaphysical books. For two hours, while my wife was shopping, I went over every book in the section, but found nothing of interest. When my wife returned, I refused to leave until I found the right book. Immediately, I turned around and there, not even two feet away from me, was Sai Baba's picture looking directly at me. The book was *The Holy Man and the Psychiatrist* by Dr. Samuel Sandweiss. After reading it, I knew I had to go to India. Although I wanted to leave immediately, events conspired to force me to postpone the trip for six months. Excited, I left for India feeling that, even if I did not get an interview, I would work on myself by meditating and accepting whatever happened.

My first trip to the ashram in Puttaparthi was in 1977. I had made arrangements with a friend who had traveled to India before me to meet there. She was supposed to protect me from the culture shock. Unfortunately, she met me at the airport in Bangalore and told me that she was returning to the United States immediately. In semi-shock at being left alone in a strange country, I left the airport and checked into the East West Hotel in Bangalore. There I met Walt Neubauer, who was Elsie Cowan's secretary at the time. Elsie was a longtime devotee of Sathya Sai Baba. Mr. Neubauer graciously offered to share a taxi with me for the trip to Puttaparthi. I immediately checked out of the hotel and joined him for the long journey. Time passed quickly as he told me many intriguing stories and experiences with Sai Baba. He also gave me a crash course in what to expect at the ashram, as well as what was expected of me.

As there was no festival at the time, I was able to secure a room to myself. There were bars on the windows, but no glass. As I had been told to bring mosquito netting, and the room was on the second floor, I had to assume the bars would keep out only the larger mosquitoes. At that time, in 1977, the room was completely empty of any furnishings and had an Indian-style toilet, which was a hole in the floor. The bathing area, bath, which was in the room, was separated from the rest of the room by a 4-inch ledge, which was designed to keep the water from running into the main part of the room. The only running water was a faucet approximately two feet off the ground in the enclosed "bathing area." One showered with cold water by soaping up and dumping a bucket of water on oneself. As there was a constant drip from the faucet, extremely large roaches playing in the bath area inhabited the room. Fortunately, I had approached my trip with the proper attitude. I had decided before leaving home that I would work on myself, meditate as often as possible, and accept whatever happened. I was told that, if the accommodations did not meet my expectations, then it was time to review my expectations. With this attitude, I settled into my room, thankful that I was by myself and not sharing the room with seven other people as I had been told might happen. I rapidly unpacked, set up my sleeping bag and mosquito netting, and excitedly rushed down to evening darshan.

The evening was dark and cloudy, with impending thunderstorms. As I waited for my first sight of the avatar, huge black birds began squawking loudly, completely filling the air so that no sky was visible. I was reminded of the story of Arjuna, the famous archer of the *Bhagavad Gita*, who fired arrows over the heads of a crowd of people to protect them from injury from above. It is said that he completely filled the air with arrows so that no harm came to the people. It seemed to me that millions of birds had completely blocked out the sky; the noise from their squawking was deafening. To this day, I've never observed a similar phenomenon. Simultaneously, Sai Baba appeared at the edge of the porch. As rain was imminent, He merely waved and returned inside. I returned to my room feeling happy and prepared for the night. While roaches skittered around behind their ledge, I made a pact with them that they would stay near the dripping water and not interrupt my sleep on the floor in my sleeping bag. I rapidly fell asleep.

I rose early the next morning determined to adjust to life in the ashram as soon as possible. I resolved to stay firm in my conviction of accepting whatever happened. Wandering alone in the ashram, I was amazed that the bustle and activity seen the previous evening had completely disappeared. In its stead was an empty calm. I approached someone, asked if he spoke English, and inquired what time darshan was. He replied, "Swami has left for Bangalore." Everyone had gone with Him, including my new friend, Walt Neubauer. (Later, Walt told me he had known Sai Baba was leaving in the morning, but was under strict orders not to inform anyone.) Now what? I was completely alone in a foreign country; all the taxi drivers had left, taking devotees back to Whitefield to be with Swami. Only the ashram residents remained. With a sigh, I reviewed my policy on acceptance, and set out to find a taxi driver. I was able to send a message to Bangalore, and then waited for a taxi to come and pick me up. This was definitely a lesson in acceptance.

After accepting the idea of staying in a sleeping bag on the floor, alternately fighting mosquitoes and large roaches while listening to the drip, drip, drip of water, I found myself staying in a luxurious hotel with running water, a shower, and excellent food. In addition, the crowds at Whitefield were much smaller than those in Puttaparthi, and I was almost always in the first row at darshan. I managed to make two good friends, one who shared a taxi with me on the trips to Whitefield from Bangalore; the other was a traveling sadhu. I have learned much about spirituality and satsang from the two of them. I vividly recall one darshan at Whitefield. I was sitting between my two friends meditating, waiting for Swami's arrival. When He came out, He seemed to float as He walked. When He passed us, there was a loud whoosh, which was both audible and palpable. In amazement, I turned to my sadhu friend, who had been traveling in India for seven years, and said, "Did you feel that?" He smiled and calmly said, "Of course; when He does that, you can't miss it," as if this were an everyday experience. It seemed as if Swami was confirming His omnipotent powers just for me.

During this trip, I met several doctors and asked them if they had witnessed any miracles. The first physician was a young man who had been educated at Swami's school. He told me of a young man in his early twenties who had severe rheumatoid arthritis. This crippling disease had so affected this individual that he was constantly in a wheelchair, unable to walk or even sit more than 20 minutes without pain. He had been to physicians all over the world, but none had been able to help. As a last resort, he came to Swami. When the time came to be called for an interview, the young physician was outside Swami's room, along with the patient and his father. Swami beckoned for him to come in. The father bent down to pick the boy up from the wheelchair, as it was necessary to carry him everywhere. As he did so, Swami said, "No, help him walk." With the help of the doctor on one side and the father on the other, it took the boy about 20 minutes to walk across the short veranda. The doctor waited outside to help him back into his wheelchair. To his amazement, when the interview was finished, the boy came out walking perfectly normally, folded up his wheelchair and carried it away.

Dr. Rajeswari, the obstetrician-gynecologist who was the head of the Bangalore hospital, told me the following story. A patient of hers was scheduled for a hysterectomy for fibroid tumors. On the doctor's rounds the morning of the surgery, the patient told her that Swami had come during the night, ripped out a fleshy mass of tissue, and told her she did not need surgery. Dr. Rajeswari was skeptical, but when she pulled back the sheet to examine the patient, there was a healed scar present that had not been there the day before. On further examination, the tumor had completely disappeared and the uterus was back to normal.

A few days before my departure, I was thinking about my friend who was supposed to have met me when I arrived in India. She had told me a story about Indra Devi, an old devotee of Swami's and a well-known yoga teacher. Evidently, Indra Devi complained to Swami that she was constantly running out of the vibhuti that He made for her, because she was giving it to others. Swami tapped the little vibhuti box and told her it would never be empty again - and it never was; it constantly refilled itself. When I heard this, I thought, "It would be great to have something like that." Then I thought, "No, it would be better if the power was in my hands; then it would never run out, and I would always have it with me." Then I promptly forgot about this.

My last day for an interview came. I had not been called. Swami was winding His way back and forth between the men and women's lines. When He was directly across from me, I realized I had missed my chance to speak to Him, because He would then continue His serpentine pattern, which would pass me by. However, He made a 180-degree turn and walked directly up to me. I clasped my hands together in supplication and asked Him for permission to leave. To my surprise, He bent over, clasped both my hands in His, and said, "Yes, yes, yes." There is no doubt in my mind that He was answering my prayer of a few days before. As if to confirm this, after darshan a crowd gathered around me and asked me what had happened. They, too, knew something special had occurred.

On my third trip to India, while waiting in the darshan line, a book about Swami that I was reading intrigued the man next to me. Specifically, he was enthralled by the beautiful picture on the cover. I was finished with the book, so I offered it to him as a gift. He then told me an incredible story. Approximately five years earlier, he had a family with a one-year-old son. Over a fairly short period of time, this man began to lose his eyesight. When he was almost blind, he decided to kill himself by jumping out of a multi-story building. He was alone in the room when, just as he was ready to jump, an arm appeared out of nowhere and grabbed him. A voice said, "What are you doing? You have much to live for." He began to argue with the voice saying, "What do I have to live for? I am going blind." The voice answered, "What about your wife and son?" He was then instructed to go to Puttaparthi to see Sai Baba, whom he had never heard of.

While he was waiting in the line for darshan, Sai Baba approached him and told him he had a brain tumor but that he was not to worry because he would be cured. Swami then materialized vibhuti for him and told him to eat it. His vision slowly began to improve, and when he regained his sight, he became a permanent resident of the ashram. About two years later, his vision again began to deteriorate again. Swami again saw him, told him that the tumor was growing, and squeezed his head saying, "Now the tumor will shrink." The man said that he could feel his head getting smaller. His vision returned completely.

While returning from one of my recent trips to India, I met an Indian man who told me his sister's story. She was a devotee of Sai Baba. While she was in the hospital in India suffering from a bleeding ulcer, her doctor ordered milk to be given through a tube going into her stomach. However, the nurse misunderstood the order and hooked the milk up to the intravenous line. The doctor did not discover the mistake until the second bottle was being given. This should have killed her. But, while the milk was running, his sister had a visit from Sai Baba who told her she would be fine. She was transferred to the intensive-care unit and had no untoward side-effects from the IV milk.

During the times I visited with Dr. Rajeswari at the hospital, she told many stories about Swami. One of my favorites shows Swami's omniscience, empathy and humor while, at the same time, giving instruction and guidance. The hospital at Whitefield had been established approximately 13 years earlier. They still did not have running water for the hospital, and so it had to be hauled for the operating rooms and patients' general maintenance, as well as for other necessities. This was a great hardship. One day Dr. Rajeswari approached Swami to ask Him about obtaining running water. She felt she had been very patient while six wells had been drilled, without one of them producing any water. She picked an area she thought would have water and then approached Swami to ask Him if she could drill there. Swami said, "Yes, yes, yes." With much enthusiasm, she made all the necessary arrangements to drill the well. Everyone involved was very surprised when it was dry. She angrily confronted Swami, as a loving mother to a disobedient son, and told him the well was dry. His reply was "What did you expect? There is no water there." She responded, "But Swami, you told me I could drill there." He lovingly answered, "You asked me if you could drill there, and I said yes." Then He looked at her and said, "Everything comes in its own time." Within two months, she was contacted by the World Health Organization. They told her that they had reviewed the situation, decided the hospital was a worthy project, and sent their engineers to determine where to drill the well. They paid for everything. Of course, today the hospital has water.

The most amazing story Dr. Rajeswari shared with me was her experience of being brought back from the dead. She had not been feeling well for several days, suffering from chest pain and dizziness. She informed Swami, and He told her He would take care of her. However, He told her to make sure that she saw a doctor to get her hypertension under control. Being a busy physician, she failed to take Swami's advice. She suffered a fatal heart attack. When she arrived at the small hospital emergency room, the EKG showed ventricular fibrillation, an extreme condition where the heart is not functioning, requiring electroshock therapy to bring it back to its normal rhythm. She emphasized that it was not ventricular tachycardia, a condition that sometimes spontaneously reverses, but ventricular fibrillation. As they did not have the personnel or the equipment where she was being treated, they tried to transfer her to a larger hospital. However, her heart stopped. They later told her that she had died on the way to the other hospital. During that time, she was unconscious and has no memory of what happened. When she awoke in the hospital, the entire room was orange. Everywhere she looked she saw orange. She said to the nurse, "I have been in many hospitals all over the world, but I have never seen a hospital room that was orange." The nurse replied, "Are you crazy, woman? There is no orange here." She said she later checked the EKG for herself and confirmed the presence of ventricular fibrillation.

One often hears that when you visit the ashram, you should ask Swami's permission to leave. I put this off to the many rumors you hear when embarking on a journey to Puttaparthi. That was until Dr. Rajeswari told me what happened to her. At the time, she was married and had a busy medical practice in India. She was visiting Whitefield (the ashram in Bangalore) and, on the day she was leaving, she dutifully asked Swami for permission. His answer stunned her: "You can't leave; you are going to run my hospital!" "But Swami," she replied, "You don't have a hospital!" That was in May. By August there was a hospital. Needless to say, she remained there in dharmic service until her death many years later. Swami has now built a state-of-the-art hospital in Puttaparthi and, at present, another one is being constructed at Whitefield. These hospitals serve everyone free of charge.

I myself have operated on patients who said they saw Sai Baba in the operating room before their surgery. One such lady, who I was operating on years later for a different condition said, before she was anesthetized, "The last time you operated on me, Sai Baba was here." I had completely forgotten.

It has been my practice for many years to talk about spiritual matters to my patients when I feel they are open to it. I have a picture of Sai Baba on my desk, which was a gift from Him on my first trip. It is a black-and-white photo, and many of my patients ask if the picture is of Johnny Mathis or Charley Pride.

On one lady's first visit to my office, she mentioned she was going to India. I immediately told her to stop and see Sai Baba in Puttaparthi; it would be worth the extra trip. As she did not seem very interested in this, I immediately dropped it and forgot about it. Three months later she called and told me she felt she should go to India to see Sai Baba as, not only I, but another friend as well, had told her to do so. She then told me the following story.

This same friend was in a hospital in Scottsdale, Arizona, dying from ovarian cancer. A doctor came and informed her he had been asked to be a consultant in her case. He touched her abdomen, and she immediately felt better. He told her she would be fine. Then he left. The next day, when her doctor visited her, she thanked him for asking the other doctor to consult with him. Her doctor said, "I did not ask anyone to see you in consultation. What did he look like?" When she told him that it had been a short, black man in an orange gown with an Afro, he said, "We have no one on staff who looks like that." Several weeks later, while visiting a friend, she saw a picture of Sai Baba and realized He was the one who came to the hospital and made her feel better. It was then that she found out about Sai Baba. Apparently, she is still in remission.

Over the years, I have found it necessary to call on Swami numerous times. One of the most urgent of those calls regarded a patient who came to my office with an acute surgical abdomen. My examination revealed a patient with acute abdominal pain who was near shock from intra-abdominal blood loss. She thought she had aborted spontaneously a month ago and had even had a D & C then, but the exam showed a live, four-month fetus with a normal fetal heart. When I informed her she needed immediate surgery, she began to cry. I misunderstood this for fear and assured her everything would be all right. She said, "You don't understand; everyone has been telling me this was in my head." She had seen 11 doctors in the last month, visiting various emergency rooms at different times. By the time I had started the emergency surgery, she was in shock from intra-abdominal blood loss despite our giving her blood transfusions. On opening the abdomen, it was filled with blood; each time we sponged, it would rapidly refill faster than we could empty it! I realized she had an abdominal pregnancy, with a living fetus that could not survive. The placenta was implanted on the sacrum, bleeding from all areas with no way to stop it. (An abdominal pregnancy is the most serious type of ectopic pregnancy; usually they occur in the tube, but this one had occurred at the junction of the uterus and tube. It was implanted involving the ovary, subsequently spreading to the pelvis. There is no way for the fetus to survive.) By this time, the anesthesiologist was telling me that her blood pressure was zero. I silently asked Swami for help and rapidly proceeded to perform a hysterectomy as she was bleeding from the uterus and ovary where the pregnancy had originally been. I had no choice, even though the patient was only 26 years old; this was now a life-saving procedure. I was no longer concerned with her fertility, but her life. Her blood pressure stabilized, and we were finally able to get ahead of the bleeding and get her under control. The postoperative course was completely uneventful, and she left the hospital on the third day.

On one of her post-op visits, she told me of her experience. At the time when she had no blood pressure, she left her body and was above us watching. She told me everything that had occurred, and said she realized she was dying. She said she knew we had saved her life, and she was given a choice whether to leave her body permanently, but decided not to. Swami's hand is always there. Whenever I get into trouble, I ask him for advice. Obviously, in the operating room I ask a little more urgently for His help, especially in a case where there is an emergency or where the situation is getting out of hand. He has never failed to assist me, guide me, and keep me out of trouble. When things are going well, and before every surgery, I dedicate my actions to Him.

In my medical practice, as well as everyday living, I try to make my life His message. He has taught me patience, humility, wisdom, and the realization that I am not the doer. I always try to follow His teachings. Some important things I've learned:

Love all, serve all.

Do not work for the fruits of your actions.

See God everywhere and in everyone at all times.

The solution to every problem is absorption in God-consciousness.

Remembering the name of God is the only thing one needs to do in this Kali Yuga.

I received some advice from Dr. John Hislop, whom I consider myself lucky to have known: We should constantly hold Swami's hand, no matter what we are doing; and it is easier to remember God if we say "Sai Ram" silently to ourselves whenever we see someone else in passing.

Of course, I have encountered a lot of skepticism from colleagues and other individuals when I talk about Swami. I can only state what I have experienced, and I do not worry about their opinion. Hopefully, I can sow a little seed in their minds that they may some day follow up on. Being one of the founding members of the American Holistic Medical Association, I have long been interested in treating the body, mind, and spirit. Swami has blessed me with untold gifts, not the least of which have been my patients. He has given me the privilege to care for them, and the wisdom to treat not only their bodies but also their minds, while always encouraging them to pursue the spiritual path.

Over the years, since I have been with Swami, I have learned to be more patient and more compassionate; I have left behind the prejudice I was raised with. I do not judge, and this has helped my patients open up to me. I have more fun with my patients now. Even though they are coming to see me with problems, often embarrassing ones, most now enjoy coming to see me. We have a special rapport and, generally, they leave having enjoyed the visit (even though I am a gynecologist). I have learned to handle problem patients, or patients with problems that are not physical. Previously, I would find that depressed patients would also leave me depressed, as they dumped all their problems on me. Now, merely by silently repeating my mantra while I am sitting and listening to them, I find that their problems seem to disappear. I am able to remain calm, and they leave with some of their burden lifted. And I am doing nothing but silently repeating Om Sai Ram.

We can all be gurus, since a guru is nothing more than a teacher. When someone you know is having a problem, just listen. Frequently they just need a sounding board. How many times have you heard people say, "Strangers just come up and tell me their problems, even when I'm standing in line at the grocery store"? They think they have some special gift. Well, the gift is they are willing to listen! Everyone wants to tell you about their troubles and, if you are a good listener, you can do seva for them. And if you are being affected by their problems, just silently repeat God's name to yourself; you will be surprised at the result.

There is some advice I would give to Swami devotees, especially those in America. There is a tendency for people who consider themselves spiritual seekers to pursue many different paths. Instead of sticking with one, they proceed from one thing to another. Sai Baba gives the analogy of digging a well in one place, going down

15 feet, and saying there's no water there. They then proceed to dig many shallow wells and never obtain water. It is much better to stick with one well until we obtain what we are looking for. Let us not forget that the avatar is present among us; we are extremely fortunate to be born in this age and to know Sai Baba. It is a mistake, a grave mistake, to think there is something better out there and continue looking for it when all the time it is directly in front of us.

What has Sai Baba meant to me? How often do I call for His help during surgery? I have thought deeply about this while writing this chapter. I realize I call on Him almost constantly, since all surgeries are a little bit complicated. Recently I returned from India, having taken my son for his first visit. My goal has been for all my children to see Swami, and this was the last one. I needed to put the finishing touches on this chapter, but I couldn't seem to complete it.

After returning from our trip, the surgeries that I performed seemed to get more difficult each time. My last one was a hysterectomy on a short, very obese patient (more than 300 pounds) who had extremely heavy bleeding, so much so that she needed blood transfusions on two different occasions in the last year. While hysterectomy was recommended, no other surgeon seemed willing to do it because of the technical difficulty involved in surgery for a patient of that size. Her very enlarged uterus, which could not move up or down, would make the surgery much more difficult. It was a surgical and anesthetic nightmare.

When I saw her for the first time, she had just bled down to a hemoglobin of 6 gms (normal is 12-14) and had just been seen in the emergency room. She was finally convinced she needed something done. After stopping the bleeding with hormones and treating her with medications to improve her blood count prior to surgery, I scheduled her for surgery. The surgery was the nightmare I thought it would be. It was almost impossible to see anything due to the amount of intra-abdominal fat and the enlarged and fixed uterus. She hemorrhaged from the uterine artery and lost a great deal of blood, which required multiple transfusions. Needless to say, I asked Swami for help before, during, and after surgery. I began to wonder where He was. Actually, I knew He was there but was wondering what He was doing.

After we finished the operation, we were far behind in our transfusions and fluid replacement. However, the IV had infiltrated, and all attempts at IVs and arterial lines by many anesthesiologists failed, again because of her extreme weight. I found myself in the intensive care unit with a patient who had no urine output, was very pale, and obviously blood-depleted. I had no way to give her blood or fluids. Her pulse rate was extremely high, and her blood pressure very low. Every physician we called for help seemed to be busy with his or her own problems. The general surgeon I usually call was at her mother's funeral! We could not even turn the patient from side to side in the bed, because she filled the entire bed and could not be turned.

What to do? I began saying the Gayatri mantra on my japamala. I realized I was not the doer, only the witness. I wondered if the patient would die. When I was about halfway through my japamala, my spouse called me and asked if I had tried vibhuti. She volunteered to bring some. I was very surprised to realize that she had thought of the vibhuti and I had not. While saying the Gayatri, and on hearing about the vibhuti, I realized what Sai is to my life. He **is** my life. Not only my life, but it seems I have trained my family the same way.

I continued to say the Gayatri. Suddenly, the anesthesiologist got an arterial line in after about 180 sticks in the neck. We gave the patient blood and fluids, and she slowly responded. She left the hospital just the other day in good condition.

One of the many things Swami has taught me is that the solution to every problem is absorption in God-consciousness. It has saved me many times, and I am sure will continue to do so. I have found that whenever I am confronted with any problem, I take a deep breath and think of God. Suddenly, all difficulties disappear; it is just like a trip to Sai's ashram in India, where the world melts away and one finds the inner Self where there is only One.

Health is the essential prerequisite for success in all aspects of life and for realizing the four ideals that should guide humans, namely: moral living, prosperity (of the spirit), fulfilling beneficial desires and liberation from grief. Everywhere man seeks to live happily and peacefully, but happiness and peacefulness are not won from worldly activities. The body that yearns to be happy and secure is subject to disease, decay and death. However, the Indweller, the Self, within the body is not born nor does it die. It is the Atma, God; the body is the temple of God. Hence, it is the duty of man to keep the temple in good condition.

Sathya Sai Baba
Sathya Sai Speaks, Vol. XI, p 148

Bhagavan & the Cardiac Surgeon
Choudary Voleti, M. D.

Health and education must be free to all mankind.

Although I was born in the same state, Andhra Pradesh, in the small town of Chittor, merely a hundred miles away from Sathya Sai Baba's ashram in Puttaparthi, I was not aware of Bhagavan for the first fifty years of my life. It is the unique hospital appropriately named Sri Sathya Sai Institute of Higher Medical Sciences that brought me into His fold.

My father decided my fate when, with good intentions, he opted for me to go to medical school, though my original intention was to become an engineer. After I entered medical school, I decided to become a cardiac surgeon. As there were few training programs for cardiac surgery in India, I joined the bandwagon of Indian doctors migrating to the Promise Land, to the good old United States of America. With God's grace and hard work, I was able to finish my cardiac surgery training and establish myself in the field of cardiac surgery, first in New York City, and later, in Los Angeles.

I come from a very religious family and had a strong belief in God. I thank my parents immensely for instilling this attitude in me from an early age. Though I was very successful in my life, both professionally and personally, I was still restless and confused and lacked any sense of inner peace. I was also constantly aware of the lack of health care available to the average Indian. The prevalence of heart diseases in India and their aggressiveness, which afflict all strata of society, always made me look for avenues that I could embark upon to serve the Indian population. I attended several international meetings, which gave me a good grasp of the progress in cardiac surgery all over the world. It also gave me a chance to follow the progress of health care and, especially, cardiac surgery in India. Though I was thrilled to see cardiac surgery being established in India, it was disappointing to realize that it had quickly become a commercial product available only to the few who were well placed in society. Though I made several trips back to India in the eighties to perform cardiac surgery, I was quickly disenchanted by the practice of catering to the rich. I was deeply affected by not being able to help the poor and desperate in India who were suffering from the ravages of heart disease.

Everyone, once he comes into Bhagavan's fold, realizes two things: nothing happens without His blessings, and everything happens in its own time. When I heard about this unique hospital, providing modern medical care in heart, kidney and eye diseases to everyone, free of charge irrespective of cast, color and creed, I was both fascinated and elated. Fascinated that expensive cardiac surgical care could be provided free in India, and elated because this was an avenue where I could give service to the Indian people. I was so involved in the hospital itself that I did not even have a clue about the divine hand that was behind all of this.

My first impression of the hospital, built in a pristine rural setting of about one hundred and five acres, was one of utter disbelief. The building looked more like an architectural monument than a mere hospital. It is well known that the first impression a patient has about a hospital goes a long way in helping him develop a positive attitude.

Bhagavan proclaimed in November 1990, during His 65th birthday celebration, that a super specialty hospital would be built in exactly one year's time. True to the divine command, the three hundred thousand square foot Sri Sathya Sai Institute of Higher Medical Sciences, sometimes referred to as the Super Specialty Hospital, was built in exactly one year. On the first day, not one but four open-heart surgery procedures were successfully performed. It took fifteen architects five months to finish the plans and, during the remaining seven months, an Indian construction company actually completed the construction work. I am part of a user group in Los Angeles and have been involved with the planning of a tertiary medical center very similar to the Super Specialty Hospital. It took us three years just to have the plans finalized. In any industrialized country, it would normally take seven years to build a similar hospital.

Apart from the grounds, which are kept very clean, the first thing that attracts you to the hospital is the overwhelming beauty and uniqueness of its external appearance. The building represents a singular combination of form and function expressed by its beauty and strength. The central dome is the chest, and the two wings on either side are the two arms of Bhagavan physically embracing and spiritually absolving patients, families, visitors, and employees alike.

The first room one enters is the prayer hall located inside the central dome. Only the spiritually overwhelming granite statue of Lord Vinayaka overshadows the sheer size and spectacular beauty of this room. The peaceful ethereal ambiance in this room pervades the entire hospital. Apart from the clean well-ventilated corridors, the lack of clutter and confusion associated with a specialty hospital is obvious at every step. The two wings on either side house the three specialties and their support structures. All the departments are equipped with ultramodern facilities equal to any advanced hospital in the world. This is the divine paradox: it is modern and sophisticated, yet it is free.

Bhagavan's hospital is setting an example by providing health services of the highest standard along with a sense of spiritual dedication to the poor. No expense was spared in equipping each department. The modern nature of the equipment is only rivaled by the single-minded work ethics of the employees. It is very clear that, in spite of the diverse linguistic and geographical background of the employees in the hospital, their common thread is their zeal to practice Bhagavan's teachings:

Hands that help are holier than the lips that pray.

The secret of happiness is not in what one likes to do but liking what one has to do.

Know that I am always with you, prompting you and guiding you.

Live always in that constant presence.

The director of the hospital, Dr. Safaya, who has been with the hospital project from the very beginning, rightfully calls this a "temple of healing." The patient receives treatment for his illness but, at the same time, his mind and spirit also receive treatment. Patients feel that they have been given a new lease on life, and they develop a renewed purpose in living. The hospital is constructed utilizing natural ventilation to minimize the energy requirements. The quality of care provided to the patients is exceptional, and the results are comparable to any leading hospital in the world. I strongly believe that the ever-present invisible divine hand guides all the employees. When I saw the hospital and the facilities available, I realized that it was a dream come true. I could at last fulfill my life's desire to help my less fortunate countrymen.

During my first visit to Puttaparthi, I had the rare opportunity of having an interview with Bhagavan. When I humbly requested His permission to be able to provide my services in the hospital, His kind reply was that it was my hospital and that I could freely work there. That gave me the inspiration I needed to start recruiting a network of healthcare professionals who were experienced in providing care to patients with various cardiac problems. Just by asking, I was able to enlist people who had never even heard of Bhagavan and had never visited India. I soon realized the common bond uniting the team was the spirit of selfless service to their fellow man.

Over the past five years, we were able to form a network of Cardiologists, Cardiac Surgeons, Cardiac Anesthesiologists and allied health care personnel involved in heart diseases from all over the United States. We have been able to visit and work in Bhagavan's hospital periodically several times a year. The team's main intention is to mesh with the existing personnel in the hospital and work as an extended team sharing ideas and improving each other's knowledge. Each trip of mine is more fulfilling than the previous one, both with respect to attaining my desire to serve the poor as well as in strengthening my own spirituality.

As soon as I return to Los Angeles, even before my jet lag is over, I start preparing for my next trip. During my stay in Puttaparthi, Bhagavan arranges my daily schedule, fulfilling both my personal and spiritual needs. His darshan in the morning is always a rejuvenating experience. When work has kept me from attending the evening darshan and bhajan, He kindly remarks, *Duty comes before devotion.* Except when I get some specific instructions from Bhagavan, I have no idea of the actual patient whom I will be helping. In the spirit of service, the identity of the patient never seems to matter.

One of the most impressive aspects to serving in the hospital is the zeal and selfless service rendered by the employees. I consider myself very fortunate to be part of this spirit of service. In the beginning, it was interesting to see that not all the employees, especially some of the physicians, were devotees of Bhagavan. They came to work in the hospital for various personal reasons. But their dedication to work and concern for the well-being of the patients seemed to be as intense as the rest of the employees who were Bhagavan's devotees. But as time went by, every person working in the hospital became an ardent Sathya Sai Baba devotee.

I had personally experienced the unwavering commitment of these chosen people. One of my visits to the hospital happened to be during the last week of March. After the Shivaratri celebrations in late February, Bhagavan left Puttaparthi, His "work place," to go to Brindavan in Bangalore, His "home." Normally, work permitting, all the employees look forward eagerly to Bhagavan's darshan and bhajans at least once a day. However, during these last ten days of March, I came to see the single-minded, selfless service rendered by the hospital employees under the most trying circumstances. Without Bhagavan, the entire ashram is like a ghost town. The temperature was soaring every day to over 110 degrees. The desert heat becomes oppressive even prior to dawn and after dusk when one would expect some relief. The sweltering heat relentlessly pervades the living quarters. The only air-conditioned place is the hospital. The welcome relief is at least three months away when Bhagavan returns and the monsoons begin. During this period, the hospital still functions to its full capacity oblivious to all these adversities.

I could not work for more than nine days. I was physically exhausted and spiritually drained. However, I saw that all the employees of the hospital were maintaining their usual calm composure and carrying on their full load of work. Their unwavering faith in Bhagavan and their spirit of service to the underprivileged seemed to carry them through these testing times.

Of course, a few fortunate employees, who have both the time and the means, travel to Brindavan for Bhagavan's darshan and bhajans. The hospital employees resort to unique ways of keeping themselves occupied and entertained in the evenings. One evening, they performed a variety program consisting of a bhajan contest and fashion show put on by all the children of the hospital employees. Needless to say, the quality of the program was very high and original. I was even more surprised when they told me that the program had not been rehearsed, and yet every move fell into place as if it had been repeatedly rehearsed and orchestrated. To me, this clearly shows their sincerity as well as the often unseen phenomena of Bhagavan's invisible hand, the divine conductor.

During one of my visits, I was able to be part of Bhagavan's divine leela. One morning, He took me to a very healthy looking young man in his late thirties and instructed me to perform heart surgery. As soon as I went to the hospital, I looked for his medical information in the computer. Not only had he not had a single test performed, but no other doctor had seen him. After all his tests were completed, including an angiogram, we saw that all his major heart arteries were significantly blocked. He underwent an uneventful four-vessel bypass. Since then, there have been many more mind-boggling instances where Bhagavan has intervened for His devotees just in the nick of time. One morning, during darshan, I asked Bhagavan about His interventions in saving His devotee's lives and wondered what my perplexing role was in all these leelas. He replied, *The surgeon is as good as His instrument.*

The number of Bhagavan's "old students" working in the hospital seems to be increasing every year. It seems as if all of them perform beyond their job descriptions and go out of the way to make sure all aspects of the hospital run smoothly. During one of my many visits, the students working in the hospital decided to organize a Health Exhibition. Many of them worked day and night, and a handful of them worked for a straight thirty-six-hour period in order to meet the deadline. When the work was completed, it was a spectacular presentation, which enabled the public to see all aspects of medicine. Bhagavan opened the fair. The various disease patterns were highlighted through picture posters and actual models of body parts. The presentation's well-deserved emphasis was on prevention. One could walk through the model of the heart following the actual flow of blood through that organ. This helped the visitor understand the function of heart. Similar presentations were displayed for diseases of the eyes and kidney.

Bhagavan is a medical enigma. For the last 55 years, He has weighed the same 108 pounds, no more or less. His blood pressure has always been normal, 110/70, without any physiological fluctuations associated with age or emotional states. I had an occasion to check Bhagavan's pulse a couple of months ago. It was a steady 63 beat per minute. Even as He is approaching 75 years, there is not a single physiological change. His hair is still thick, black and curly. He still reads even the small print without the help of eyeglasses. Nobody has ever seen Him sleep. He survives on 300 calories per day. For mere existence, without any physical activity, the body needs 10 calories per pound per day. In spite of consuming only 300 calories per day, Bhagavan works from dawn to dusk and dusk to dawn. I was so perplexed with this that I asked Him how anybody could survive on 300 calories. His simple reply was that we consume energy and He creates energy. During the health fair, when the Chief of Ophthalmology routinely examined Bhagavan's eyes, he was shocked to find that His eyes were like those of a teenager without any of the changes that age normally produces in the lens or the retina.

When Bhagavan sustained a hip fracture, to the utter disbelief of the physicians, He was walking around during darshan three days later. Normally, it would take four to five weeks for mere mortals to stand on a fractured leg. When I approached Him about all these physiological aberrations, He said that it is all a matter of mind over body. He also said that His divine powers are only for mankind, and He never uses them for His own personal benefit.

Bhagavan instructs people to not eat meat or consume alcohol and to refrain from smoking. His advice is to eat vegetarian food in moderation. *Do not live to eat but eat to live.* One day, He was explaining how an Indian bread cooked over fire has only 70 calories, but the same bread fried in oil has 170 calories. He was also explaining how we should all drink at least six glasses of water every day to compensate for the loss of fluids from perspiration, breathing and urine. He was explaining the ravages of high cholesterol, as well as the causes for high blood pressure and strokes. The extent and depth of His medical knowledge is astounding. During our heart team's first interview, He talked so much about heart surgery that we were all amazed. He told us how the first open-heart surgery, using a heart lung machine, was successfully performed in 1953. He also explained to our heart-lung machine technician the importance of the connections and how he should be very careful about air bubbles in the circuit. These are details familiar only to people who interact with these machines day in and day out.

Bhagavan feels that mind and doctors cause 90% of diseases. The stress of so-called civilized society causes the majority of diseases, such as high blood pressure, anxiety syndromes, and the least understood one, chronic fatigue syndrome. One of my Pathology books says, "The sorrow which has no vent in tears makes other organs weep." The medical community is fully aware of the ravages of the emerging new bacterial strains that are not sensitive to currently available antibiotics. This scenario has emerged from indiscriminate use of antibiotics. As Bhagavan said, it is the mind and the physicians that are the cause for the majority of diseases affecting mankind today. There are many avenues one can follow to achieve stress reduction. My approach has always been simple and practical. Do the best you can under the circumstances and leave the rest to the Lord. He will always help the needy. Meditation and Yoga are two other very effective practices for relief of stress.

By profession, I belong to a very special group of surgeons who deal with serious life-threatening medical situations. After a while, it is not unusual for us to succumb to pride and ego and become first-class prima donnas. As the popular story goes, how many cardiac surgeons does it take to screw in a light bulb? The answer is very simple, one cardiac surgeon. All he has to do is to hold the bulb, and it will screw in by itself; that is because the whole world revolves around him. For a long time I, too, had an inflated ego and a false sense of reality. Since I have come into Bhagavan's fold, I have realized the falsehood and frailty of the cardiac surgeon. It took me a few trips to Puttaparthi and a few interviews with Bhagavan to realize the age-old axiom, "Man cuts and God heals." I realize that I have to do the best I am capable of, and God will do the rest.

My trip to Puttaparthi in July 1999 was an excellent example of putting things in perspective. As soon as I make up my mind and fix the dates for the Puttaparthi trip, I can never rest or relax until I see Bhagavan. The feeling becomes more pressing when I board the aircraft in Los Angeles. This time I was lucky to fly straight into Bangalore avoiding not only a nine-hour layover in Singapore, but also bypassing Madras. This trip was more exciting, as I was privileged to know ahead of time that Bhagavan was planning to build another specialty hospital in Bangalore, and I was actually going to see the site selected by Him. Also, a visit during Guru Pournima is always a genuine reason to be excited. It was 1:00 p.m. by the time I had seen the beautiful site for the future hospital in the desirable suburbs of Bangalore. After a nerve racking two-hour drive, we reached the ashram. It took a few minutes to freshen up, and then, on the way to darshan, I heard the celestial music in the Poornachandra Hall start playing. With my heart pounding I rushed in, my eyes frantically searching for Bhagavan. The next thing I knew, I was looking at His radiant, smiling face. Immediately, I fell at His feet to avail myself of a satisfying padnamaskar. When I finally got up, He was kind enough to inquire briefly about my trip, and then He proceeded to glide away. That brief encounter was the experience I had been dreaming of since I left home. Only He can make things like these cherished encounters happen so smoothly, as if they have been practiced and rehearsed many times before.

After bhajans, sung by His students, and so spiritually satisfying, we were invited into His quarters. The architect's model of the new hospital was breathtaking in its beauty and strength. He talked to us about the details of the project. He asked us to sit on the sofa, reminding us that we have forgotten how to sit comfortably on the floor. As the meeting came to an end, we were getting up from the sofa in front of Bhagavan and, impulsively, extended our hands to help Him get up. His immediate response was that the hands we were giving were for us only, and that He does not need our hands to help Him. To our utter amazement, and before we were aware of what was happening, He was already on His feet, and His hands were above ours gently lifting us. As we were leaving, Bhagavan asked me to see a patient in the hospital.

This particular patient happens to be a long time devotee who is completely surrendered to Bhagavan. The patient has been running a home and school for disabled and orphaned children in Africa for the last two decades. Three years ago, during one of Bhagavan's evening discourses, he collapsed and was without pulse or blood pressure, and Bhagavan successfully revived him. He remained healthy for three years and continued his service to handicapped children. During his present visit to Puttaparthi, he was making arrangements to fly back home when Bhagavan instructed him to cancel his trip and get admitted to the hospital. When they completed all the tests, the doctors realized that he had serious blockages in all three important arteries of his heart, and he had to undergo bypass surgery in order to survive. They also realized that, due to Bhagavan's intervention, he had survived a fatal heart attack three years ago. After the tests were performed, Bhagavan actually visited the patient in the hospital and assured him that his operation would be performed successfully by me. I learned all these details by speaking to the patient and the doctors involved.

The next morning, during darshan, I told Bhagavan that the patient needed surgery and, as in prior cases, Bhagavan fixed Thursday morning for surgery. He also told me that He would come to the hospital to see the patient in the evening. When the hospital opened, Bhagavan used to visit every week, but for the last five years, His visits have been very infrequent, once every six months or so. I know very well the excitement and enthusiasm that is created in anticipation of even a rumor that Bhagavan is likely to visit. I also know that even Bhagavan's shadow cannot predict His next move. Having all this in mind, I was careful to share this information only with the patient and the director of the hospital. Tuesday morning, at 10 a.m., there was such excitement in the cardiac suite that it took me a couple of minutes to realize that Bhagavan had arrived and was heading to the patient's room. He spent almost ten minutes reassuring and comforting His devotee. It was an emotional scene, Bhagavan pouring out the love of a thousand mothers, and the patient so moved and overwhelmed with His love.

Thursday morning at 7 a.m., during darshan, Bhagavan asked me at what time the operation was scheduled. I told Him we would start around 9:00 a.m., and the actual operation would begin by 9.30 a.m. He told me not to wait until 9:00 but to start immediately. I realized, long ago, not to question or try to comprehend Bhagavan but to follow His instructions. Without waiting for darshan, I gathered the team and rushed to the hospital. As soon as the patient arrived in the operating room, I asked him what was going on. He confessed that the whole night he was having chest pains. I asked him if he informed the nurse or the doctor on duty. His sincere reply was that he prayed to Bhagavan. With the kind of blockages this patient had, severe chest pain would indicate an impending fatal heart attack. It was then that I realized that waiting until 9:30 to start this operation would have been fatal. The operation went well, and the patient recovered uneventfully. That afternoon, when I mentioned to Bhagavan these details, my utter inability to understand Him, and expressed my mental state of confusion and despair, His only reply was His brilliant all-knowing smile.

We work six days a week, and Sunday is generally a day of rest where there is time to do personal errands, make telephone calls and, reluctantly, reestablish contact with the outside world. That Sunday, I was not feeling completely well, still recovering from jet lag and also my myalgias were bothering me. I wanted to tell Bhagavan about my daughter's engagement. During darshan, I was fortunate to get His attention and requested to talk to Him. He promptly took the cardiac anesthesiologist and me into the interview room. It was a rare privilege to have Bhagavan's attention just for us. He asked us about our children. With eagerness and enthusiasm, I told Him about my daughter's engagement. He approved the date set for the marriage and reassured me everything was going to go well. He asked, *What does the boy do?* "He is a lawyer," I told Him. Remembering that my daughter was also a lawyer, Bhagavan's immediate jocular response was, *Then they can have a court of law at home.*

He talked about the new hospital and details about the time frame. Then, with a twinkle in His eye, He asked us about the operations for the day. We mildly protested that it was Sunday and the operating theater was closed. At this juncture, He invited us to His quarters for "tiffin" at noontime. We were so excited. As we were getting up to leave, He gave us a beautiful piece of cloth with specific instructions to get a safari suite made and wear it for Guru Pournima. The series of surprises are not over yet. He came out with an envelope with six crisp hundred-rupee notes to cover the tailor's charges. By this time, I was so overwhelmed with His love and attention that I started crying. His blessing for my daughter's wedding relieved me of a massive weight off my back. His awesome attention about my myalgias reassured me that nothing was seriously wrong with me except my wild imagination. His kind actions relieved my anxiety about my health as well as what to wear for Guru Pournima. This was a staggering experience, to say the least. This is the kind of love only He can shower you with; a thousand mothers and fathers cannot even come close.

We found the right tailor, even though he did not have a sign outside his shop. The ritual of taking measurements was painlessly over and, though it was Sunday, he promised to deliver everything by Tuesday evening. The only problem I had was that he only charged us 300 rupees and Bhagavan had given us 600.

Promptly at 11:55 a.m., we were at His quarters. The students, who also act as security guards, took us inside. It is a totally unnerving experience to be in His quarters. You are so enveloped with excitement and confusion that, for a while, you are totally lost. The quarters were very clean, with every piece of furniture in its place, and it was very quiet. It is Bhagavan's amazing love and attention to even the minutest detail, such as where you sit and your personal needs, that brings you back to your senses. After we regained our stability, He invited us into the dining hall. There was a beautiful table, that can seat a dozen people, filled with about fifteen freshly made vegetarian dishes. We had to eat all the dishes without complaining, and He only took three spoonfuls. All the time, He was making sure that the students were attending to all our needs, and we were pampered with attention.

From 12:30 to 1:50 p.m., He talked to us on subjects varying from astronomy to zoology. His instruction to us on dharana, which is the fundamental basis for meditation, was very timely. He told us the early morning hours between 3 a.m. to 5 a.m. are the best for meditation. One needs a comfortable mat to sit on and an isolated corner, far from the daily noise, is ideal. In the beginning, a light source is essential to maintain concentration, until one can achieve the state of control over the monkey mind. Sitting with a straight back is of paramount importance. The essence of meditation is the entire process of breathing. The respiratory cycle consists of inhalation, holding the breath, followed by expiration. The duration of expiration should be equal to or, if possible, longer than inhalation. Repeating "So Hum" is the ultimate integrating feature. He told us something very important. He said that the rate of respiration is inversely proportional to the life span. For instance, birds and dogs have the fastest respiratory rate and, therefore, have the shortest life span.

He explained to us, at length, about faith. Bhagavan said faith is the solid foundation on which one builds love. Love leads one to truth, and truth is none other than God. So, a life that is filled with faith ends in bliss. When we were ready to leave after this rare enlightening experience, He gave us another piece of cloth, for a second suit to be made, telling us that it was a better brand. That explained the extra three hundred-rupees! This is proof that everything Bhagavan does has a purpose, however inconsequential it may appear, and every word that comes out of His mouth is truth.

During this last trip, the day after I performed surgery on Bhagavan's devotee, the cardiac anesthesiologist mentioned that he had seen many surgeons operate. He told me he was very impressed, because he had never seen another surgeon look at Bhagavan's picture on the wall in the operating room, momentarily close his eyes, and then make the skin incision. We all have algorithms for our surgical techniques and, since I have entered into Bhagavan's sphere, this has been mine.

As soon as I return from my trips to Bhagavan, I get ready to make another trip, always worrying about the poor people in India. One time, when I mentioned this to Bhagavan, He told me that all patients are alike, and the service I perform is the same whether it is done in America or India.

I want to conclude with the amazing and powerful encounters of my last trip to Bhagavan in February and March 2000. As I alluded to earlier, each of my trips to Bhagavan seem to be more fulfilling than the previous ones. But this experience will stand out singularly in my heart and mind for the rest of my life and reverberate in my soul forever.

Three of us from the US, Dr. Thumati, a cardiologist, Dr. Bareddy, a cardiac anesthesiologist, and I were sitting in darshan waiting eagerly for Bhagavan's blessing to start our work at the hospital. The soothing celestial music commenced and Bhagavan glided into the darshan hall. As usual, He was materializing vibhuti for some, giving padnamaskar to others and choosing fortunate devotees for interviews. Though one is used to this routine every day, on the first day of each trip, the wait seems eternal until Bhagavan steps onto the veranda. Finally, when we saw His divine smile of recognition, we were elated. Responding to our ecstasy, He said, *The Thrimurthis are here.* What a powerful designation! (The Thrimurthis refer to the 3 most powerful aspects of divinity, namely Brahma the creator, Vishnu the preserver and Shiva the destroyer.) He specifically instructed us to look up a certain patient and perform a diagnosis on him. The patient had blockages in all three arteries and needed major heart surgery. After work, we went back to the ashram and sat down on the veranda. As soon as we arrived, the Vice-Chancellor came out of the interview room and said Swami wanted to see us. This was most perplexing because everybody knows there are no windows to look out on to the veranda and see who is sitting there. In spite of this, the minute we sat down, the Vice-Chancellor came out with this message.

An invitation like this always creates excitement and perplexity. With joy and palpitations, we sat at Bhagavan's feet. Dr.Thumati told Him that the patient He had asked us to see needed multiple bypass surgery, adding that the patient was willing to, unhesitatingly, follow Swami's recommendation. Swami said, *Yes, patient is a good man, but his wife is very worried and anxious.* He said He would talk to the patient's wife and son, and that we should arrange for surgery on Wednesday which was an auspicious day.

As we were getting ready to start work at the hospital, the news of Swami's arrival spread like wildfire. I knew right away that He was coming to see the patient. I went straight to the patient's room and, sure enough, Swami arrived with the administrative staff. The patient was absolutely surprised at this unexpected visit and his rare good fortune. He was overwhelmed and could not control his tears of happiness. Swami spent fifteen minutes talking to us about the details of the surgery and, at the same time, reassuring and blessing the patient. Swami then said something that really opened my eyes. He told the patient, *This is your prapthi and My duty.* It is difficult to translate the word "prapthi;" it can only be explained as "what one deserves or what one has earned." With that powerful revelation, He materialized vibhuti for the patient and left the room. His parting words were even more perplexing for a casual observer. He told the patient how lucky he was that the three specialists he needed had arrived from United States just in time for his operation.

To the utter delight and surprise of the staff, He toured the whole surgical suite making kind remarks and permitting people to have long awaited padnamaskarams. After work that afternoon, we were able to attend darshan. While we were waiting on the veranda for the bhajans to begin, to our delight Swami took us into the interview room and talked to us for almost thirty minutes. Most of His remarks concerned the new hospital in Bangalore. It was fascinating to feel the infectious enthusiasm of Bhagavan whenever he talked about the new hospital. He also gave us some insight into the friendly competitive attitude of the two neighboring states for Swami's high profile humanitarian projects.

I then told Swami that my friend's wife was concerned that He was loosing weight. After telling us what a great devotee she has been, He said she was wrong. He has been feeling great and had not lost any weight. It is always fascinating to see Swami being defensive during discussions, and this time was no exception. After saying He had not lost any weight and felt fine, He looked at Dr.Thumati and, as if looking for support, asked him for his opinion. Dr.Thumati earnestly replied, "Yes Swami, You look like you are loosing weight." Showing much disappointment on His face and mild irritation in His voice, He countered, *You are a very good doctor but you are wrong, I am the same 108 pounds for the last sixty years.* Having said that, His face lit up with a mischievous smile. Within a few moments, we experienced His humor, mock anger and child like divinity. I will remember and cherish these privileged private encounters forever.

While I was waiting for darshan on the day of the surgery, Swami came and asked, *Why are you still here?* "Swami, I need your darshan before starting surgery." *Okay, go start the surgery early.* It took us about five hours to do the four bypasses. As per protocol, I sent word to Bhagavan that surgery had gone well, and the patient was doing fine.

The afternoon darshan turned out to be memorable and thrilling – memorable for the sequence of events and thrilling for the unexpected nature of the experience. As soon as I sat down on the veranda, the secretary came to me and said that Swami was looking for me. No sooner had he finished saying this than Swami came out of the interview room straight to me and said, *Perfect operation, four bypasses.* All I could do was nod my head, as words deserted me. Then to make my life both difficult and delightful at the same time, He walked around the whole veranda talking to everybody about the operation. I was so overwhelmed and in pure ecstasy when He proceeded to announce to everybody, *Swami is very, very, very happy.* That alone has made my life worthwhile.

The next morning in darshan, I told Swami that the breathing tube had been removed and the patient was progressing very well except for some high blood pressure. Swami said, *Don't worry about the high blood pressure as it is related to his age.* This is what we normally see in older patients after cardiac surgery. Later, when we went to the hospital to see the patient, he looked very stable, with excellent vital signs and no complaints. Although the patient looked excellent, the chest x-ray was disturbing with some evidence of blood collection around the heart. However, since we had tubes in the area draining the blood, it did not bother me very much.

During the afternoon bhajans, Swami, again, inquired about the patient. We told Him he was doing well and had been sitting in a chair for a while. That made Him very happy. Then, He looked at me and asked if He should go and see the patient now or in the morning. As it was really none of my business, I mumbled, "Maybe now, Swami, as it may be a little quieter now than in the morning." Even before I had finished my mumbling, He said that He would go and visit the patient in the morning and disappeared inside the interview room.

After a couple of minutes, Swami came out, and one of His boys started sprinting like an arrow across the hall towards His quarters. Swami walked towards Dr.Thumati and me and said, *One of you sit in the back and the other in the front.* As we started walking towards the center of the hall, we saw the red colored BMW majestically rolling between the rows of female devotees. Swami sat in the back behind the driver; I sat next to Him; Dr.Thumati sat in the front seat. Sitting next to Bhagavan, with only the armrest between us, was the most unnerving feeling. Then, added to this, there was the smell inside the car; it was so fragrant and soothing that it was beyond comprehension. The car slowly started rolling towards the gate on to the main street. The minute the car turned into the main street, there was a sea of humanity lining the street on both sides. I asked Bhagavan, "How on earth can so many people in such a short time know about Your trip? With a twinkle in His eye, He said, *Sir, this is faster than your television.* The mass of people lining the street all the way to the hospital were of all colors, creeds and nationalities.

They were so happy and excited to see Swami; their faces lit up with big spontaneous smiles. I have never seen so many people so happy. They were throwing flowers and garlands on the car; they were lighting incense and breaking coconuts. I was so moved that I started crying helplessly. During the car ride, He talked to us about many topics ranging from the *Vedas* to Einstein.

We approached the entrance to the hospital where there was a red carpet rolled out, and Swami's cart was ready and waiting. Swami and Dr.Safaya sat in the front, and Dr. Thumati and I sat in the back. The cart was driven straight up to the surgical suite where everybody was ready. The patient could not believe his good fortune. Swami talked to him very sweetly, reassuring him that he was making excellent progress and telling him that he should follow the doctor's instructions. Swami blessed the staff all along the ramp and, as we reached the front door, His car was ready with the door open. Swami got in through the open door, and Dr.Thumati sat in the front. I sat in the back realizing, to my utter consternation, that I was sitting behind the driver now, where Swami had been sitting before. With that revelation, there was no way I could relax or put things into perspective. Again, on the way back, there was the same spectacle of masses of people showing their veneration for Bhagavan. As we were approaching the observatory, I heard the roar of an elephant reverberating in my ears. This brought me partially to my senses. The car came to a stop, and Swami rolled down His window to greet Sai Gita. Acknowledging her Master, she let out another deafening roar. I was still crying, not realizing if this was really happening or a dream. The car rolled gently in to the darshan hall between thousands of devotees sitting and waiting Swami's arrival. I then realized that on that particular day it had been exactly seven years since I had first visited the ashram and had my first darshan of Swami. I had always had this fascination with taking a ride with Swami in His car but, even in my wildest dreams, I did not think it would be possible. The entire trip took about thirty minutes. Those thirty minutes transported me to a different world that, previously, had existed only in my wildest imaginings. Now, in reality, I had experienced how Swami can make so many people happy and content in such a short time. With all these emotions my head started spinning; I was losing my perspective on reality. As soon as the car stopped, I got out and prostrated at Swami's feet. He was kind and understanding enough to give me the few moments needed to gather myself together and not let this divine experience cloud my emotions and unsettle my senses.

At a practical level, I was still concerned with the patient's progress. There was still x-ray evidence of blood collecting around the heart. Through sheer confusion, the junior staff at the hospital totally misunderstood my orders and removed the tube around the heart instead of the tube around the lung. I was hoping that the tube around the heart would drain the excess blood collection. Now, even that hope had vanished. Remembering that Swami had proclaimed that this was a perfect operation, the only recourse I had that night was to pray to Swami to correct the problem. The next morning, after another x-ray had been taken, it was absolutely normal. For the scientists and the doubting Thomas's, the x-rays are still there for verification.

Saturday morning was Shivaratri and the darshan hall was overflowing with devotees. Darshan was very beautiful with a festive atmosphere. Swami suddenly stopped in front of me and said, *Bring the patient at 6 pm, no, bring him at 5 pm.* "Bring the patient to afternoon darshan Swami?" *Yes.* "How am I going to bring him in this massive crowd, Swami?" *In My car.* "Where should I make him sit, Swami?" He pointed to the corner closest to His seat and said the patient could sit there in a chair. From past experience, I have learned to ask Swami for exact instructions, and I was certainly happy that I did. We checked the patient in the hospital, and he was doing very well. But I still was not clear why Swami wanted the patient to be brought to the darshan hall with the hundreds of thousands in the Shivaratri crowd. The patient gave me the answer. Apparently, he slept well until six am. When he woke up, he realized that it was Shivaratri, and he began to relentlessly pray to Swami for His darshan on this holy day.

It was only two years ago that this patient came into Swami's orbit. All his life he had been a very religious person. His communication with God was by namasmarana: chanting the

Lord's name constantly. Last December, when he retired from active duty, he asked Swami for permission to work permanently in the ashram. To his surprise, Swami asked him to take care of his health and then he could work in the ashram. This surprised this otherwise very healthy active person. However, he decided to take care of the only medical problem that he was aware of, an ear discharge from chronic infection. When he went to consult the ear specialist, he was subjected to a battery of tests in preparation for an ear operation. To everybody's surprise, this very healthy looking person failed his tests, and the angiogram showed life threatening blockages in his heart. That, to me, is a concrete example of the power of namasmarana.

When I returned to the guesthouse, the secretary was on the telephone. He had a strange message for me from Swami. Swami wanted a 100% guarantee from me that, from a medical point of view, the patient would tolerate the trip to the ashram that afternoon. As I had gone on this route with Swami before, I told the secretary to tell Swami that I gave a 100% guarantee, knowing full well this was just a test for me and had nothing to do with the patient.

We performed major open-heart surgery on Wednesday; on Thursday, the patient sat in a chair; on Friday, he walked about three hundred yards. Now, on Saturday, he made a trip to the ashram in his street clothes looking like any other devotee. During His Shivaratri discourse, Swami told the huge audience how lucky this gentlemen was; how just in time, it so happened, three specialists had come from America to take care of him. This is a perfect example of a divine leela.

Before I was absorbed into Bhagavan's fold, my life was chaotic; it was like sailing through uncharted waters. Now, I can sense a feeling of calm and balance in my personal and professional life, which brings new meaning and purpose to my existence. Whatever I am doing, Bhagavan is always in the back of my mind guiding me at every step. Whether there is pleasure or pain, grief or happiness, I live and breathe Bhagavan's loving presence all the time.

Geriatric Sai-chiatry
Jonathan Lieff, M.D.

The constant presence of Swami in my life and His guiding hand in my medical practice have been abundantly evident. It seems to me that there have been so many blessings, and so many funny coincidences, which saved me at the last second, that these must be from Him. So many troubles and difficulties have been overcome without any control from me other than faith in Him, that I believe He has been guiding me for many years.

I believe that the blessings of my college and medical school education at Harvard and Yale, and all my medical positions, have been direct gifts from Swami. My spiritual vision, my experiences of the atma, and the peace that comes from contemplation on Swami, have become more and more the major focus of my life.

At Yale College, I majored in religion, mathematics and, finally, pre-medicine. Since my graduation from Harvard Medical School and residency in psychiatry, my specialty has been in geriatric psychiatry, or neuropsychiatry - that is, the treatment of patients who have combined medical, neurological and psychiatric illnesses. A large percent of patients have been elderly, with a smaller percent brain injured or medically ill younger people. My role in our treatment teams is directing the team and, specifically, using psychotropic medications with these ill patients.

Since there was no field called geriatric psychiatry when I began to practice medicine in 1972, I have had the opportunity to start a number of different types of programs that later became accepted. At present, I am medical director of a system that provides services for approximately 300 nursing homes and four hospital units. My own function in this organization is to supervise the psychiatric, psychological and nursing staff who travel to the nursing homes to treat the patients, and to treat the most ill of the patients myself. These include patients who are very medically ill and very agitated, or who do not eat, as well as psychiatric patients who can be combative, violent or suicidal. We also treat many handicapped and neurologically injured patients who have additional medical and psychiatric illnesses.

When I started out in medicine in the early seventies, I was drawn to the Eastern or integrative style of medicine and had created several programs attempting to integrate Western medicine with Chinese medicine, Ayurvedic medicine, and Shaman medicine traditions. I was very interested in the use of meditation, vegetarian diet, and healing arts in the practice of medicine. Prior to graduation from medical school, I was involved in developing several eclectic healing centers including weekend workshops and weekly meditation classes. At that time, I was somewhat radical in my belief in the use of these meditative and healing practices and was somewhat skeptical about conventional psychopharmacology. To this day, I believe strongly in the usefulness of all of those techniques. But, it certainly was not clear in the 1970's that I would later become president of a Western subspecialty organization and direct a large hospital program specializing in Western psychotropic medications. It was an experience in Brindavan in 1978 that changed the way I would practice medicine.

Although I had some sort of unconscious awareness of Sathya Sai Baba before the spring of 1977, I didn't connect the visions of His face that were appearing in my meditation until I was about to leave on a trip to Vancouver in May 1977. After meditating for ten years in a variety of ways, and being involved for those ten years in teaching meditation classes, both in the hospitals and in Sufi dance classes, I found I was spiritually adrift. I had become disillusioned with the many different gurus whom I had met in my search for a teacher and master of yoga. Although I had already started to develop geriatric programs, I was still searching, two years out of my psychiatric residency, for my niche in my profession. My prejudices at that time were toward the Eastern healing traditions and against aggressive psycho-pharmacology.

For a number of years I had helped direct a satsang where many different teachers came to teach. I was also a leader in a musical group that provided backup music for some of these traveling gurus and for Sufi dance classes. Our sixteen piece musical group was invited to perform at a major United Nations Conference on Human Settlements in Vancouver. We were to perform music of the world religions as an entertainment backdrop for the United Nations' conference. We played an eclectic mix of music based on religious prayers and mantras in the styles of gospel jazz, reggae, and rock and roll. This opportunity occurred in a strange way. I had been working as a healer and was able to help a British man named Patrick who worked for the United Nations and was suffering from a severe case of Parkinson's disorder with tremor and shuffling gait. He had traveled unsuccessfully to other healers around the world looking for a cure for his Parkinson's, and he was brought to me to attempt a healing. Patrick's job was organizing the Conference on Human Settlements for the United Nations. He was very inspired by our healing practice and wanted our band to perform at his conference.

The night before we left on this very unusual trip, I came upon the "Psychic Film Festival" in a movie theater in Kenmore Square in Boston. On impulse I went to the festival, which consisted of a number of brief films including the first Richard Bock film about Sathya Sai Baba. It was during this film that I first realized that it was Sathya Sai Baba's face that seemed somehow familiar to me, and I finally realized He had been the image in my meditation. I was transfixed by seeing Swami for the first time and very excited, but I didn't know what to do or where to go to find information about Him. The next day, just before leaving, I found one Indian clothing store that had one book, *Sathya Sai Speaks, Volume I,* so I took this book on my trip. It was on the plane flying to Vancouver that I first read Swami's writing. It was during this remarkable once in a lifetime trip to the UN Conference on Human Settlements that I first kept thinking about Swami. The trip was an unqualified success. Our band never played as well as they did during that time. We were able to play music for thousands of people, singing spiritual songs of the world religions.

The storekeeper had told me about a small group of four people that met to discuss Sai Baba's teaching. This was the beginning of the Brookline Sai Baba Center, near Boston, that later met at my house from 1984 to 1994. At that time, I had never been to India and had never really thought of going, but when the small group announced that they were going to see Swami at Christmas time, I told them I was coming too.

In December of 1977, the five members of our center went to see Swami. I was extremely excited and didn't know what to expect. I was reading Dr. Sandweiss's book *Sai Baba, The Holy Man and The Psychiatrist* at the time. Certainly many readers know about the uncertainty and the unusual leelas that are often part of trips to see Swami. Sandweiss's book captures the difficult and interesting trip during the seventies.

I couldn't sleep the night before I first saw Baba. We were in the darshan line early and were near the front. Of course, there weren't many people then. The first time I saw Him in person, Swami walked up to me and said, *I'll see you tomorrow.* I, of course, took the meaning of tomorrow in my time scale rather than in His. The next day he ignored me completely, and I was devastated. Several days later, He came up to me again and said, *You go up and down, don't do that; don't worry. I'll see you tomorrow.* I was only slightly more able to deal with this statement the second time. The rest of this first glorious trip included a time when I sat very near Swami at a wedding, and when I was right near His foot for a discourse about Jesus at the Christmas dinner. And then we returned to Boston.

My appetite had just been whetted at this point. I yearned constantly to go back to see Him as soon as possible. The next opportunity was in the following spring when I found out that he was giving his thirty-day Summer Showers Course in Brindavan just outside of Bangalore. I heard that this was a course for Indian students but that Americans might be able to sit in also. I had no idea what was in store for me when I left for six weeks in the spring of 1978. When I arrived at the college, prior to the course, someone announced that some Westerners could take the full course and live in the hostel. This was a dream come true. I signed up immediately and was given a room with two other Americans students. This was a strange situation, taking a college course and, at the same time, living in an ashram in India. We were sleeping on the floor, getting up long before dawn, going to a strenuous Iyengar-style Hatha yoga course, working hard all day until Swami's discourse and bhajans each night. However, back in the room, we had a competitive academic atmosphere just like Medical School. We went to the lectures each day on the varieties of religious experiences and then attended the evening discourses from Swami, largely on the *Bhagavata*, including detailed tales about Krishna and the gopis. When Swami walked back from the hall to His house, several times He passed right near us.

Towards the end of the thirty days, we were allowed to take the examinations with the boys. We received diplomas directly from Swami's hand. But the most wonderful part of this examination was that two Westerners were given a plaque by Swami for scoring so well. We two were allowed to go up to the stage and take padnamaskar as Swami handed us the plaques. Someone was snapping pictures at this exact moment, and these photos have been on my altar ever since. These photographs have sustained me in times of trouble.

Many things happened that summer that have had a lasting impact on my life. I will only focus on four specific events that are relevant to my medical practice. Each Sunday there were no lectures, and Swami would take us in trucks to a village to do service. We were loaded onto trucks with brooms and bags, and we would all fan out and clean one of the villages. At the end of several hours' work, the village looked beautiful, and Swami would come and give us ice cream. This experience made an indelible imprint on my brain of how a village, in several hours, could be changed from a filthy, unhealthy place into a beautiful Shangri La.

The second event was a sudden unexpected visit by Swami to the hostel to look at our rooms. One day during afternoon siesta, we heard that Swami was in the hostel looking around. We all ran down the corridor to see Swami in a bedroom watching two students from America, one massaging the other. I could hear Swami's sweet voice say, *No, this is not the way. Here...* and He held out his hand and made vibhuti for the two Americans. It struck me that Swami was emphasizing the importance of faith in healing over the massage.

The third incident was during the lectures. Out of thirty days of daily lectures on the varieties of world religions and levels of devotion, only one lecture was about Sufism. At that time, Sufism was my primary belief system, and I had been teaching Sufi classes for ten years before this trip. It could not have been an accident that, for that one lecture about Sufism, Swami came into the auditorium and sat directly in the chair in front of me. I believe this was the only time He sat for the full lecture. His hair was right in front of me during that hour. I don't remember anything that was said during that time, as I could only concentrate on His hair right in front of my face. Swami has said that His hair is a forest, and people come there for a rest. I rested in His hair on that day and many other times since. For me, this was in some way a validation of my confused and circuitous spiritual searching for direction.

The fourth incident was the most dramatic. I believe it was this experience that greatly influenced the direction my practice was to take. In 1978, the college was not large. In fact, the tree was still in the courtyard where darshan was held. There was a quadrangle bordered by the main administrative building including the clinic in the middle, the hostel dormitory where we stayed on the left, and Swami's house on the right. The auditorium where we had classes and heard Swami's daily discourse was out of the quadrangle and down the street. Darshan occurred in the quadrangle twice each day. Swami lived in His house and His elephant, Sai Gita, lived behind.

One day, I was in my room studying during the lunch break. Suddenly, an Indian man, whom I later learned was a doctor, came running into my room and said there was a problem, and I had to come immediately. I asked him what the problem was, and he said that one of the American students was ill and needed my attention. I was very reluctant to go since I considered myself a student and not a visiting doctor. At home, I was considered somewhat radical in medicine with my interest in meditation, Sufi dance and holistic medicine. In India, I was enjoying being quite conservative and anonymous. I was just being a simple student in the school of spirituality. The rigorous and time-consuming program was very good for my soul. I felt that I didn't want to attract any attention or get involved in any unusual situations that might single me out in any way. I told the gentleman that he should find the Indian doctors on duty to help. But he would not take no for an answer and demanded that I come and evaluate this American man. He said that as an American doctor, I would be more useful for this American who was in trouble.

As we walked down the hall to the American man's room, I recalled seeing him each day as I walked past his room to and from the lectures. His behavior had seemed odd to me, because he didn't seem to be going to the classes or benefiting from Swami's course. He was always lying on his mattress staring at the ceiling. But at that time, I was not paying attention to others. Swami had said that, at his ashram, we were to be responsible for our own behavior. We were not there to socialize but to learn. Swami had said that we were not only responsible for our own behavior, but we were also responsible for any misinterpretations of our behavior by others. This had seemed strange to me, but I didn't want involvement with anything unusual so as to avoid any misinterpretations of my behavior. Swami wanted us to behave in a very respectful manner and not to offend the conservative cultural sensibilities of the Indian people around us. In a way, we seemed to be a test case for the inclusion of Westerners in the course. So, I didn't want to deal with any trouble. But as it turned out, Swami had another idea in mind.

We walked into the room of the American who was lying on his mattress staring at the ceiling. He was also a medical doctor and was a partner of a devotee in America. No one seemed to know too much about his background. He didn't really want to talk with me, but spoke begrudgingly. He was angry and appeared to be delusional. I found myself doing a psychiatric evaluation, without consent, for a man who was not my patient, in a place that was not my clinic, in a country where I knew nothing about the customs, laws, rules or medications used. I did not think I had the authority or license to practice medicine in India.

The longer we stayed, the more it seemed to me that the American doctor was psychotic. He appeared to be having hallucinations. Someone said that he had not been eating properly for days, and maybe he had an electrolyte disturbance or dehydration causing a psychotic delirium. I thought it was also possible that he had a more serious psychiatric disturbance such as schizophrenia. His history was unavailable, except for the fact that he was a doctor who had recently joined the practice of another doctor in America.

Suddenly, the man stood up and walked quickly out of the room. We were startled and stood up and followed him. After a while, I was walking quickly behind him alone. I didn't know what my responsibility was, but I knew I needed to follow him. I felt put upon to be the one who had to make a decision in this situation. This psychotic American, looking quite bizarre, was now walking out of the hostel into the quadrangle near where darshan was held. There was no darshan at this time, but there were some Indian people walking around, and they looked at him strangely. This was very disturbing to me, because they also looked strangely at me, associating me in their minds with this unusual and bizarre situation. I realized that my conservative cover was now gone.

The American then walked passed the courtyard and was heading toward Swami's house. I was the only one following behind him. It seemed as if he wanted to go and see the elephant, but I was getting worried. We were definitely not in the right place. What is striking to me now is that I was confused about what to do. On many lonely nights in charge of the psychiatric emergency service, where all kinds of violent emergencies arose, there was no question of what to do. If this man were in the emergency room, he would have been treated already. One night, several policemen brought a very violent man to the emergency room. This man tried to attack anyone who came near him including myself. He was forced to take antipsychotic medication and then locked in a secure unit. The next day, another doctor let him go. He returned to the hospital that second afternoon with a gun and shot and killed the doctor who had released him. I was trained to act and take care of dangerous situations. But to do this in Swami's courtyard? What form of healing should take place here?

The American was now at the gate of Swami's house. An elderly Indian man was guarding Swami's house and walked up to the big, angry, bizarre American and said, "No, you can't go there. Please stop." The old man put his hands gently on the large American who had crossed his arms in a pensive stance. Suddenly, the American flung his huge arms open and the old man went flying back and fell and hit his head.

"Oh my God! Wait a second!" I thought. The old man was now lying on the ground, seemingly unconscious, and the American was going behind Swami's house to see Sai Gita. I had to do something. This was out of control. I picked up the old man and carried him to the nearest medical area, which was the female clinic. Several of us then went and grabbed the American and physically brought him, against his will, to the medical area in the administrative building. The Indian doctors told me I had to treat the American now. "What medication should we give him?" They asked. Again, I was put off. "What do you mean I have to treat him? He is here in India. I don't have a license in India to dispense medications. You should treat him." I said. "How?" they asked. "He is an American and you know best what would be his treatment in America." I didn't even know what the pharmacopoeia was in India. I had no idea which medicines were available. "What medicine do you have?" I asked. They had a version of Thorazine, and we gave him an injection. He was much calmer after that.

My thoughts were confused. This was indeed a bizarre situation. I leave America, where I work in psychiatric units and give patients Thorazine, and where we search for alternative treatments that are not as toxic then, half way around the world in Swami's ashram, I am commanded to give intramuscular Thorazine. In fact, I resisted at first giving the Thorazine, even though it was the appropriate and best treatment for this situation, whether in the ashram or back in the United States in the psychiatric unit.

Just after this, we received word that Swami had given permission for the American to leave the ashram and go to the hospital. I learned that ECT (Electric Convulsion Therapy) was a very common treatment at this hospital. However, I asked them to wait and not treat him with ECT, as I thought this treatment decision should be done when he returned to America for treatment.

When I returned to the ashram, I realized that people would now associate me with this psychotic American. Even my most sincere attempts to blend in would now be difficult since many people had seen us together as I followed him through the courtyard. In fact, one of the Indian ladies pointed to me and whispered about the crazy American.

What I really learned, however, from this dramatic event is that I had not acted quickly enough to treat this dangerous man who was psychotic. In the emergency room, at the first dangerous sign, I would have given him an injection. Here I was in an ashram, far away from what I believed was my medical reality. In fact, it is very important for me to aggressively follow my intuition of when to treat patients. While in medical school, because of my interest in the alternative methods, I had been reluctant to use medications and even more reluctant to use ECT. This was really an ignorant prejudice, not based upon study of what has been helpful to patients. Medications are necessary for many patients, and ECT is actually an excellent treatment if done appropriately.

The "holistic" people, who are randomly against using medications, are no more correct than people who use treatments without thought and balance. Many psychiatric medications are now good and effective medications for many different indications. But it is still not possible to scientifically determine which of the medications should be given. It is essential that judgment be used. It can be called clinical experience or intuition. Some call it a logical algorithm of a sequence of medication trials with careful clinical observation. But if we do not aggressively treat patients, often we will not help them.

This experience at Swami's Summer Showers course has never left me. If I had responded more quickly, the old man guarding Swami's house would not have been hurt. As it turned out, by the next day the old man was doing well in a bed at the ashram hospital. Swami visited him and made him vibhuti. Later that summer, I was at a meeting in Puttaparthi where Swami spoke to the Americans before we left. At this meeting, I sat just at His feet in great bliss. Swami had certainly not been angry with me for this event, but I never again forgot that my job is to be aware of patients, to be vigilant and act as quickly as is reasonable in treatment.

As the years have passed, one of the hallmarks of my program is that I am sent patients who are very resistant to many treatments. It is important that we never give up trying to help them. No matter how many difficulties arise, we must try to continue to find the newest and best medication combinations. When there is no hope, then we continue to try to be of emotional and spiritual help as well.

One patient, a young woman about twenty-five, had been attempting to kill herself for years because of persistent depression accompanied by constant suicidal thoughts. She had injured herself to the point of partial paralysis and had been living at a rehabilitation center for several years. Every psychotropic medicine known at that time had been tried on her. Her loving parents were tortured by the conflict of wanting to allow her some freedom so that she could have some quality of life even in the center where she was constantly under some type of surveillance. Yet, they knew she had to be watched because of her intermittent suicide attempts that had been pervasive and quite dangerous for years. We constantly were attempting trials of treatment with new medications and then combinations of medication. Finally, after three years of trials, a bizarre soup of five different medications worked. The suicidal ideation stopped, and she was no longer depressed. It was a very unorthodox mix of medicines and, therefore, easy for others to criticize. Whenever other doctors, who did not know the details of her multiple medication trials, saw the unusual mix, they started to lower one of the medications. Each time she immediately deteriorated into depression with suicidal thoughts. After several years, she knew enough not to allow any changes of this unusual mixture. It seems she needed this exact, very unanticipated, combination which we had found through great persistence. She eventually left the inpatient setting where she had been for more than five years. Three years after she left, she sent me a letter thanking me for persisting in trying different combinations of medications until we found one that worked. She said she now had her life back and was grateful. This was also Swami's lesson - to never give up trying to help.

Another result of this experience with Swami is that I can no longer drive by an accident without stopping. This need to stop and help comes from the incident in Swami's ashram. On a number of occasions, I have been able to be helpful as the first medical person on the scene of an automobile accident. On one spot on Martha's Vineyard, where I live in the summer, I have stopped at two very serious accidents at the very same dangerous intersection. On both occasions, I was able to stabilize a seriously injured person until the ambulance came. During this past summer, again I happened to observe an accident and be the first on the scene. I helped a dazed and injured woman who was being harassed by the wild, irresponsible driver who was guilty of causing the accident. In a bad two-car accident, I was able to call the ambulance on my cell telephone while, at the same time, stabilizing the head of the woman for about forty-five minutes until the ambulance arrived. In another situation, as I arrived, a drunken driver, who had hit an Asian College student on a bicycle, was inappropriately attempting to force her to stand up so he wouldn't be blamed for her injury. I was able to intervene and keep her calm and lying down until medical help and the police arrived. This later went to court, and I was able to give testimony to the District Attorney. Later, I learned that the driver of the car did not have a license and was also high on drugs at the time. Despite our constant worry about litigation, it is our duty, as trained medical people, to help wherever the help is needed.

While writing this section of the article about the imperative to treat, a colleague I had not heard from for years sent me a woman who, on and off for years, had had a severe psychotic disorder. She was a mother of two young children, a schoolteacher when not ill, who had severe bouts of psychotic illness, either bipolar or schizophrenia. She was also a devout Christian Scientist with a large extended family of Christian Scientists who had cared for her at home without medication during all of her bouts of psychosis.

On this one occasion, her husband and brother had become exhausted caring for her round the clock during a psychotic episode and, out of desperation, had sent her first to a Christian Science nursing home and then to a hospital to hold her for a day. They needed to send her children to relatives to be cared for in order to have time to set up the house to continue to treat her safely at home with prayer and close observation. She was now being kept in the hospital against her will. Her family wanted me to evaluate her and help them get her back to the family.

My evaluation showed that she was indeed psychotic; and certainly under any other circumstances, I would have strongly recommended medication. However, I found her husband and brother to be very sincere, loving and committed to their "no medicine" philosophy. While I totally disagreed with them and said as much, I could only respect their total sincerity and commitment to their religious belief as well as their hard work in caring for her for years. In between these bouts, I was told she was a totally normal, loving mother and teacher. Previously, I had always had a prejudice against Christian Science but, because of their strong belief, I found myself in court fighting to defend them against the wishes of the doctors at the hospital. I was able to convince the judge to release the woman to her family for treatment. When she was released to her loving family, I was moved to tears.

On a number of occasions, there have been difficulties that have damaged my hospital and nursing home programs. Over the past twenty years, these programs were on the brink of disaster more times than I would like to remember. During each of these crises, the people who worked for me looked to me for help. The problems included the closing of hospital units, the bankruptcy of a hospital, the loss of referred patients, the loss of business, the intrusion on quality of care by HMOs, the cutting of services by Medicare and Medicaid, and various forms of harassment. For some reason, we have survived each of these problems and have come out successfully on hundreds of crises over the twenty-five years.

Those around me have always thought that, as a leader and medical director of these programs, I had something to do with averting these crises. But in actual fact, my only power in any of these situations has been to pray to Swami. Because my anxieties would delude me, there is no way that I could have continued to have the level of responsibility that I have today without Swami's daily help.

One example occurred in a hospital where we had a program for more than ten years. This hospital unit had been the mainstay of our practice, and we needed it to survive. The hospital was doing very poorly financially for a variety of reasons unrelated to our unit. Knowing that the hospital was near bankruptcy, I was investigating the possibility of other hospitals taking over our geriatric psychiatry unit. But none of these plans seemed to be working. A particularly unscrupulous businessman had bought the rights to our existing hospital building. His philosophy was not to help but rather to drive the hospital out of business hoping to purchase it for a cheaper price when it was bankrupt. We were within days of extinction. In addition, certain units had to be created by Friday to meet a state legal deadline. On Thursday, the day before the fateful Friday deadline, I received three independent telephone calls from three different hospitals. Each of these hospitals offered to start a unit with one aspect of the existing unit. We hadn't even approached two of these hospitals previously. Instead of collapsing, on that same Thursday we agreed to establish three new units, each with a slight difference, that could all work together. Suddenly, instead of one unit, we had three. Eventually, these units became a much superior model for our practice. These three were a medical evaluation unit, a locked psychiatric unit, and a long-stay medical psychiatry unit. These units have now been quite successful for five years; we are just opening a fourth. It is very hard for me to believe that such a strange coincidence could happen. I can only thank Swami for another one of his manifestations.

I would like to describe another miracle that does not relate to my medical practice but was very dramatic and symbolic of the type of help that Swami has given on many occasions. Unless one has visited the Bombay airport in the middle of the night, no one would believe the absurdity and grace of what happened. On the return trip from Puttaparthi two years ago, two of us were at the Centaur Hotel in Bombay at 11 p.m. Our flight was at 3:00 in the morning, seemingly plenty of time for the five minute drive to the airport terminal. We decided to go early since anything can happen at the Bombay airport. As the cab approached the building, all we could see was what looked like a riot. There were hundreds of people, with carts filled with suitcases, pushing and shoving. They were all excited and angry in a large crowd near the building. The cab driver stopped as close to the door as he could, dumped our bags on the ground and left. We were standing there, in amazement, as hundreds of people were crowded around one door, each with a luggage cart, pushing in a completely mad traffic jam. When we asked someone what was going on, he said that there were three large international flights, each with hundreds of people, all leaving at the same time, and the airport had locked all the doors of the building but one. Everyone was trying to get into that one door. We tried to be calm, but we realized that there was no way to get into the building to get a cart, and we couldn't carry all of our luggage without one. If we waited to try to get inside and find the carts and then came out again, we would be extremely late for our flight. We were amazed and frightened by the prospect of this sudden madness.

As we stood there looking around for a clue of what to do, a very strange thing happened. A tall thin Indian man, dressed in a black suit, walked by us. I still have to ask whether we really saw this since it was so odd. But we both remember the same exact experience. This man, for some completely unknown reason, was pushing not one but two carts. As he walked by us, he dropped the two carts right in front of us and kept walking by. Neither then, nor to this day, can either of us think of any reason why a man would be wearing a suit on a hot summer night. Why would he have two empty carts at that moment when many people were clamoring to find even one? And most of all, why would he drop these two carts right in front of us?

We took the carts, put our bags on them, and started in the line to get in the door. It was still a struggle, but we were finally able to get inside and board our flight on time. We both believe that without this strange gift we would not have been able to make the flight. Once again, I have to thank Swami for His intervention. Somehow, this experience at the airport seems similar to my experience with the last minute three telephone calls that resulted in starting the hospital units. They are both so completely unlikely that they strain credibility. It is just too absurd to believe that Swami did not help. It was this type of help, on a daily basis, that has allowed our hospital programs to survive.

During the past twenty-five years, I have continued to do almost the same thing every day, that is to treat elderly patients and brain injured patients in the hospital and sub acute units. But over these years, the tone of medicine has changed. In the past ten years, there has been an increasing intrusion of the financial aspects of medicine over the clinical aspects. For many years, we were not so concerned with the amount of money that was involved in treatment, but rather were concerned about good treatment. Of course, we had to think of money in terms of having enough patients to earn a living, but we would never evaluate a patient and think of saving money rather than think of the best possible treatment. It seems very immoral to even consider saving money when there is a possibility of helping someone.

Increasingly, business competition has become an important factor in just surviving. Today, ruthless and unethical business practices have become the way of medicine in the so-called greatest teaching hospitals. The group that I work with have tried very hard to be ethical clinicians, but it has become harder and harder.

I feel one of the impacts that Swami has had on my medical practice is that I have tried, over and over, to be loyal and good to the people that I work with as well as the patients and their families. Whenever there has been a choice of a financial consideration at odds with being ethical to a colleague or helping a patient or family, we have tried not to think about the money. This loyalty among our group of colleagues has spanned organizations that were otherwise at war. Certain doctors for years have referred patients to me, and I referred them back when the treatment was completed. These referrals occurred across the lines drawn by the various corporations that claimed to own each of us.

An example occurred with one of the older, well-known doctors in my field of geriatric psychiatry. Years before, he had been annoyed with me due to competition over federal grants. I was a young upstart in the field, and both of us received major, competitive federal grants in geriatrics. He was still annoyed with me at a time when I was given an opportunity to take over his program through a secret contact from the administrator of his nursing home. Believing that ethics with a colleague were more important than the additional income I could gain, I contacted this doctor and told him what had happened. Instead of accepting the position behind his back, I described the offer to him and asked him what I should do. I explained to him that I had always respected his work and would not want to do anything to hurt him. I explained that, on several occasions, other physicians had taken programs that were mine and that I didn't want to do this to him. I told him that, since what was offered to me was already his program, I wanted to consult with him first. He thanked me for the courtesy and then said he would look into it. I lost the new position but gained the respect of a colleague. This type of situation has occurred a number of times, and each time I have tried to remember Swami and have tried to act ethically rather than in the cut-throat manner in which medicine is now being practiced in the United States.

More and more I feel the urgency to experience Swami every minute of the day. I can see the opportunity Swami gives us to practice some small spiritual part through the many interactions we have with people. Out of the approximately thirty cases that I will treat in some way each day, there are many occasions when the patients, their loved ones, or clinical staff present themselves to me in great distress. We have the choice at that moment of spending the time and energy to help and console those individuals or we can move on in the business like fashion, typical of the arrogant way of medical life in the West. We can rudely talk in front of patients as if they are objects, or we can treat even the most unconscious or demented patient with respect. I believe that Swami has said that the manner in which the doctor behaves is a good part of the treatment. In my practice, I can stop and just sit with the distraught family member, talk to the sister or daughter of my patient and just help them understand exactly what is occurring, what their options are, or just have empathy and listen to their pain.

Swami has talked about "praise and blame." Of the thirty patients each day, some group is going to praise me for great work, and some group is going to hate me, thinking I am arrogant and uncaring. Whether patients or families of patients praise or blame me usually has very little to do with anything I have done or not done. Often, they will praise me if a good result occurs by an act of God, even if I have done nothing at all to bring it about. Many times I will be accused of being uncaring in cases where, although I have spent extra time concerned about the case, there has been a negative outcome. We cannot be concerned about the praise and blame. Certainly when patients are angry and upset about something, I try to talk with them and apologize for any perceived slight, even if I didn't, in any way, do what they perceived. They may dislike me because of the bad result of the case. If I have slighted them, certainly I will apologize. I feel Swami's presence, and I believe that I must apologize for anything they might have felt from me whether I meant it or not. Any projection they might have felt of my being arrogant, or distant, or not caring enough, I must apologize for and then try to help them feel better. There are countless opportunities daily for us to love our patients and the families of our patients. What other profession would give us the opportunity of being able to console and comfort dozens of terribly distraught people each day?

All day I have the opportunity to spend the extra time and effort to love the people that are presented to me by God. This continual effort allows me to think of Swami more and more. Whenever I find myself getting nervous, worried, rushed, or angry I try to stop and think of what Swami would want, *Start the day with love, fill the day with love, end the day with love,* and *Be good, see good, do good.* This distressed person in front of me is Swami, and Swami knows exactly how I am treating him. Perhaps this attitude toward patients is our physician's mantra, our meditation, our seva, and our love. We have the opportunity to be humble and helpful all day long to distressed and ill people. God has truly given us an opportunity for sadhana.

The greatest effect that Swami has had on me as a person and as a doctor is in making me more sensitive to my patients and their families, identifying with them as if it is I who is suffering. While I can sometimes still move too quickly, I am now aware of doing this and try to slow down and listen more to everyone around me. When I make a mistake or am insensitive, I often know it instantly and pray that Swami will forgive and help me to make amends. I try to apologize immediately for any seeming insensitivity. Trying to see Swami in each person in front of me makes me search for Consciousness in old, infirm patients that might otherwise be ignored. I believe that Swami directly has sent any family member or person who has come to me. I try to sit and talk with them as long as is necessary. The greatest gift Swami has given me is that I feel glad to be alive and glad to have the opportunity to serve patients every day.

It is hard for me to write this article without mentioning two specific aspects of Swami's work that have deeply affected me. All day, every day, I am aware of the Swami's Super Specialty Hospital and the Water Project. For me, these are two of His greatest miracles. The Super Specialty Hospital is like a distant shining jewel. It gives me the understanding that medicine can be practiced in this world in the proper spiritual way. It is hard to always remember this in medicine as it is practiced in the

Western commercial rat race. Knowing about this hospital gives me courage and hope to be a real doctor. I always try to think about the proper values, even as we struggle to survive with Medicare financial problems, clinics searching for money for their job quotas and legions of Medicare officers raiding the hospitals to investigate frauds.

The Super Specialty Hospital is a shrine to the appropriate use of a hospital and has become a great inspiration for me. I wonder if there is some way to bring back the message of this hospital to the materialistic American medical system? Swami's hospital continues to grow and to glow with spirituality, volunteerism, and excellent treatment with the proper attitude. Yet, it seems that greed, materialism and unethical business practices are causing a downward spiral in American medicine. Now when dealing with the financial problems of Western medicine, I can think back to the time when I took off my sandals and prayed in the large sanctuary in the front room of the Super Specialty Hospital.

Swami has said that our behavior can have an effect on the world. I now believe that the most dramatic thing I can do is to continue to practice ethical medicine, thinking of Swami at all times. We can try in each moment to do the best action, to avoid anger, greed and the other bad qualities that Swami has taught us about. Above all, we must try to be focused on our patients and their welfare as we try to develop systems that allow this. In my case, having some administrative duties, I must figure out a way that allows the patient an appropriate amount of time for treatment. This is difficult because the insurance groups are pushing people inappropriately out of the hospital.

Ever since my experience in the Summer Showers course in 1978, the importance of volunteerism has been clear to me. It is not just a sadhana but a necessary part of society. In fact, I believe that it is only through massive volunteerism that we might be able to turn the system away from commercialism and return it to its proper values.

The second major miracle for the world is Swami's Water Project. For years, I wondered why the third world did not have clean water. Could there be something inherent in the land, the geology, or the country that does not allow clean water? Swami drilled clean wells in Puttaparthi from which He served over a million people at a time, and now he has dug clean wells for thousands of villages. The only impediment to having clean water was the will to drill the proper wells. There were problems with the government and with the lack of concern for the health of the villagers. Driving to Puttaparthi now, I see the miracle of the Sathya Sai's water tanks. This image stays with me all day as I walk through the hospital. This is a symbol for all of us, to do what is necessary for the health of the people.

Swami has given us these two miracles to inspire us in our medical practices. There is no reason for there to be bad water. There is no reason for corrupt, greedy hospitals. We should drill a good well and build a good hospital. We should build Super Specialty Hospitals around the world, and everyone must have clean water. May Swami give us the strength to help Him build this new world of medicine.

Work as Worship
Daniela Eulert-Fuchs, M. D.

The invitation to write this article came as a big surprise, a big joy and, also, a big challenge. I must admit that I have had a tendency to separate spiritual life from everyday and working life. I used to look down on my studies, thinking they were not important, until Swami showed me that He had been with me in every little detail of my academic and working life. I have heard that He once said to his students, *No shares. I want you to remember no shares.* "Swami, we promise we won't play in the stock market and get involved with any share holdings," one of the students replied. *No, no, not that,* Swami said, *No shares, no sharing, do not share God with anyone or anything. You must be 100% with God - only with God. There is no separate God-life and worldly-life. Do not separate your day into God's time and your time. You must make all your work God's work, all your time God's time.* Of course, He does not mean that we should neglect our worldly responsibilities. He says, *Do your duty in the world, engage yourself in your profession, take care of your family responsibilities, but perform all these activities in the name of God and for God's sake. Offer them all to God. That is the meaning of no shares.*

His love is the magnet that draws us closer and closer to this goal. His unspeakable sweetness is what draws us back home. I remember once sitting on a bench in the Vienna woods pondering over the essence of Baba's teachings. I had a little conversation with Him. "Please, Swamiji, tell me, what is the best sadhana? How can we reach you?" When I looked down on the ground, I saw a little string that formed the word LOVE! "Love that humbly serves Him in one of the many manifestations of His infinite Being," I thought to myself.

This was obviously also Brother Lawrence's aim, and He lets us have a taste of it in his delightful little book, *The Practice of the Presence of God.* When he began his work, he spoke to God with a filial trust in Him: "O my God, since Thou art with me, I must now, in obedience to Thy commands, apply my mind to these outward things. I beseech Thee to grant me grace to continue in Thy presence, and, to this end, prosper me with Thy assistance, receive all my works, and possess all my affections."

And later he said: "For me, the time of action does not differ from the time of prayer. In the noise and clatter of my kitchen, while several persons are together calling for many different things, I possess God in as great tranquillity as when upon my knees at the Blessed Sacrament. Sometimes, indeed, my faith becomes so clear that I almost fancy that I have lost it. The shadows which veil our vision normally seem to be fleeing away, and there begins to dawn that day which is to be without cloud and without end, the glorious day of the life to come." Brother Lawrence lived Swami's words, *Work is worship.* In our day to day working life we, too, are given the chance of spiritualizing our everyday life in order to practice and, eventually, experience the oneness of all.

When I was three years old, I remember being asked by a friend of my parents what I wanted to do later in life. Without any hesitation my answer was, "I want to become a children's doctor." Maybe, at that time, I was still connected to the knowledge about my life's plan. Later, that orientation got lost. When I was about twelve years old, I saw a film on psychoanalysis and the story of Freud, Adler and Jung. I was deeply moved and very excited. I could not sleep all night and decided that this was what I wanted to do with my life. But then in my teens, with all their ups and downs, medicine lost its appeal. Philosophy, with its questions about man's existence, arts, languages, and literature became so much more interesting. After finishing school, I burnt all my science books, absolutely convinced I would never need them again. I decided to study literature and philosophy and devote my time to music. However, this was not meant to be. Already destiny was weaving its unseen web, and little flashes shed light on the path I was to take.

In the summer, after the final examination, I had to attend classes in first aid before I could take my driving test. During one lecture, given by a doctor, I had a very strong feeling, more like an "inner calling," that medicine would have a lot to do with my life; somehow I knew that this was my path. However much I wanted to follow my inclination, I felt I could not escape my destiny.

But school was over and, in front of me, lay a long summer vacation. At that time, my parents were on a holiday in Italy, and

I went to visit them. One night, when I sat on the beach looking at the stars, a light came down towards me and, with it, came the knowledge that I had to study medicine. This "knowing" was absolutely clear, simple, and beyond doubt. This was the first time that I consciously witnessed God's guidance in my life. To everybody's astonishment, that Fall I started to study medicine. The first subject I had to study was chemistry. You can imagine how happy I was about that! Knowing there was no way around it, I, reluctantly, started studying for the exam. Maybe I would have done better if I had tried to practice one of Swami's favorite sayings: *Happiness lies not in doing what you like to do, but in liking what you have to do.*

When the day of the exam came, I had only prepared part of the required subject matter and, therefore, was quite nervous. Walking up the stairs, I met a girl I had never seen before. She was also waiting for the exam and started to explain to me one of the problems I was asked later in the test. Coming out after the exam, I felt I had not passed. I looked up to the sky and said to our dear Lord: "If it is really your will for me to practice medicine, then please let me pass this examination. I will take this as a sign from you, and I promise that, for the rest of my studies, I will be well prepared and do the utmost to please You." A few days later, when I came to the notice board to check for the results, I realized that the minimum required score had been lowered, and that I had only just passed with the minimum score. There were no longer any doubts. This was the path designed for me, and I really worked hard during the coming years.

Two years later, during the summer of 1983, my parents allowed me to go abroad for the summer. They did not grant my wish to go to India, which I had wanted to do for a long time, but told me I could go to the U.S. with a friend of mine to visit her family. At that time, I was not aware that my wish to go to India was due to a hidden longing for a spiritual path. But the Lord can come to you wherever you are; one cannot limit the Lord. In America, I met people who opened me up to the whole spiritual spectrum of India, and I felt that I had found what I had unconsciously been looking for. I studied *The Autobiography of a*

Yogi by Yogananda, Ramakrishna's *Gospel* and Vivekananda's works. When I came back home, I was already a vegetarian, interested in spiritual topics, and no longer able to fit into my group of friends.

Missing company, I prayed for satsang and was miraculously guided to an ashram led by a very remarkable lady called Guru Ananda and her adopted son, Swami Vayuananda. She had been taught by a disciple of Swami Brahmananda, the famous follower of Sri Ramakrishna Paramahansa. Being clairvoyant, she directed an ashram in Vienna where she taught Yoga and meditation. She and her adopted son had vast knowledge, as well as a library with all the ancient scriptures and works of Yogananda, Ramana Maharshi, Vivekananda and Sri Ramakrishna, to name only a few. Everything was free; we were only allowed to bring a flower or piece of fruit when we came there for lectures or meditation in the afternoons. I remember one incident clearly. She asked me if I had already worked hard for a certain exam. "Well," I said, "I have done something, but I still have a lot of time." "I am not sure," she told me, "because I was shown that the date would not be the end of July, as you think, but the twentieth of June." I didn't believe her; but one week later, I saw my name on the notice board for this exact examination date! Her comforting words gave me the courage to "Do my best and leave the rest to God." Over the remaining weeks, all went well and exactly as she had predicted.

Even though I had heard a friend mention a man in India who could perform miracles, it was in this ashram, in the spring of 1984, that I first saw a picture of Baba and heard of His true mission. One day, I looked up at His picture and silently told Him that if all that I had heard about Him was true, then I knew I would have to wait to come and see Him. I would wait until He gave me a sign that He is calling me. Two years later, I had a dream where I saw an old man whom I did not know. He was sitting on a stone at a fork in the road. His right leg was crossed over his left, and He had a piece of cloth wrapped around his head. He filled me with enormous joy and bliss. He said to me: "I am waiting for you in South India." I woke up immediately with a wonderful new feeling of bliss that stayed with me throughout the day. I knew that, even though the man in the dream didn't look like Sathya Sai Baba, this was His call. You can imagine how surprised I was to learn later that this was Shirdi Sai. The following night, again in my dream, I received detailed guidance concerning every step of my first trip to beloved Bhagavan. I saw people who would help me and those who would not, and I saw that I had to pack only hand luggage. I was shown a lot of details that later proved to be necessary.

One week later, in August 1986, my father and I were sitting on a plane bound for India. We were given crew seats because Air India had overbooked the flight. This was exactly as I had been shown in my dream. How excited I was. Already I felt as if I was coming home after a long absence.

On our way to Baba, we went on a little pilgrimage through India and had the good luck to meet Mother Theresa of Calcutta. She left a deep imprint on our hearts. The thought for the day, written on the blackboard in the motherhouse, was: "Give whatever He takes and take whatever He gives with a big smile." Every detail in the mother's surroundings carried her spirit like a signature: simple and profound.

I will never forget what she taught me. One day, she took my hand, and taking each finger separately, pronounced: "You did it to me. This is what Jesus will say one day." How deeply I felt her words. She really lived her teaching. She only preached what she practiced, and this is what made her words so precious and meaningful. "Manava seva is Madhava seva." Service to man is service to God. We, as doctors, are given the unique chance humbly to do our duty, while we are serving the Lord in our mind.

When the plane landed in Bangalore, it was as if a big weight had been lifted from my shoulders. On our trip through India, I had read *Sai Baba, The Holy Man and the Psychiatrist* by Dr. Samuel Sandweiss and could not hold back my tears. We could hardly wait to reach our final destination, Prashanti Nilayam.

Coming through the gates, I felt I had come home after a long period of exile. This was what I had waited for all my life. At that moment, I had an astonishing thought. "This moment alone, of touching this sacred earth, has been worth all the difficulties and trials of this life." The whole time with Baba was filled with so many amazing experiences that I simply stopped trying to understand what was happening to me.

One of the many remarkable things that happened during my stay with Baba was a dream He gave me. Swami was giving a lecture about C. G. Jung, the famous Swiss psychoanalyst. In the dream, I was as excited as I had been in my childhood when I had first seen the documentary of Freud, Adler, and Jung. I raised my hand and asked Swami questions that I did not understand. I found these same questions answered many years later in a biography of Jung. When I came back home after this first trip, a friend of mine, thinking I might be interested, gave me a list of Jungian psycho-analysts. This was quite extraordinary because, until recently, neither the Jungian society or the analysts were listed in the telephone book. For me, this was a confirmation to take psychoanalytical training in the Jungian school. However, many years passed until this became a reality.

Towards the end of my studies, a remarkable event occurred. I had, by accident, missed the deadline for one practical training and, because of that, I could not take my last exam in Neurology during the winter semester. I had to wait until the summer semester. This meant that I would get my degree three months later than I had planned. I was desperate. All my plans were upset. One night, Swami came into a dream and I asked Him: "When will I finish my studies?" Swami smiled, shook His head in the typical Indian way, and said: "March or May, March or May." Already, in my dream, I knew that it was going to be May. This was uncanny, because neither in person nor in dreams had He ever referred to my studies. I had never felt they mattered much. Of course, when we are in His presence, all our worldly, mundane matters seem to lose importance.

While I was preparing for this last exam, I went to a Sai retreat. During the retreat, I had a dream concerning one topic of Neurology, N. facialis. The day of the exam, a friend opened my book at random, and my eyes fell on one syndrome. It was a very infrequent disease and quite unlikely that I would be asked about it. The professor was not in the best of moods, and two colleagues that were examined before me did not pass. Then it was my turn. When the professor looked at my record of examinations, he said: "Now, let us see if she is really worth her marks." Leaning back in his chair with an expression on his face that said, "I am quite positive you won't be able to answer this," he asked: "Do you know a syndrome with Lingua plicata." "Yes," I answered and could tell him all about it, because Swami had shown it to me that same morning. You can imagine the astonishment on this man's face. I would not have known. But Swami did.

So, you can see that Swami's miraculous help with both my first and my last exam was like a beautiful frame around the years of my studies, showing me how much He had been with me through it all. After my doctorate, I went to see Swami in India and, instead of staying for three weeks as had been planned, I stayed approximately one and a half years for "higher studies." Swami often refers to Puttaparthi as a spiritual university so, after worldly scientific training, I now hoped to deepen my spiritual studies. At this time, I thought I would never work again in my profession. Since I always felt I was not attached to this work anyway, it was fine with me.

Then everything changed. Swami made it clear that I should go back to the West and do my duty. When I came back to India with my parents, we were called for an interview. When Swami asked me what I was doing, I could not answer. He was patient. In a second interview, He asked me again. Still feeling quite uncomfortable, I said: "I am a doctor." He said: *No, no, you are patient. God is doctor of doctors.* What a teaching! It really does not matter what we do. We are all in His divine clinic to cure us from ignorance and bondage. He alone can prescribe the right medicine. All that we are given to do should be done in the right spirit as a means to bring us closer to Him. The veil of ignorance must fall away so His light can reveal our true identity. Swami tells us that, in this yuga, it is appropriate to live our life in society. *Hands in society, head in the forest,* He says.

In another interview I asked Swami which specialty I should go into. He looked at me and said: "Do ladies specialty or children." While He was saying this, I felt that He meant children.

I knew that Swami never says a word without reason. When things looked desperate in finding a job, He took a lot of pressure off of me by leaving me a second alternative.

In Austria, the situation for young doctors is quite difficult. There are far too many doctors for only a few postings. After one finishes studying, one is put on a wait-list for approximately 3 years before one can start the "turnus" – a three and a half-year training for general or family practice. During this time, one works in the different departments like Gynecology, Internal Medicine, Surgery or Pediatrics and, if lucky enough, one gets the chance to specialize. When I worked in Pediatrics, I applied for this specialty but was refused, because I did not agree to do things that were not in harmony with dharma. Things looked quite desperate for me, but I knew that the puppet master, behind the scenes, was the only powerful person, and His will would prevail.

I was finally accepted at the University clinic, working in intensive care for children. This was a very difficult time. Only the thought that these little ones, in so much pain, were working out their own way towards God could pacify and console me a little bit. Later, I changed back to the department where I had been refused earlier. I had received a letter of apology and was offered training in pediatrics. During the following years, when I was feeling burdened with responsibility, working in difficult situations where I felt I did not have enough training or knowledge, Swami continuously showed me how much He was with me.

He never left me alone in difficult situations. He was always present and helped me to make the right decision. I remember once in the very beginning of my training, I was called to the gynecological department in the middle of the night for an emergency cesarean section. The woman had serious complications during labor, what we call prolapse of the cord. On my way to the department of obstetrics, I played the tape on which Swami sings the Gayatri. This had been my habit, and I prayed fervently for Him to act through me. When the baby was born, it showed no vital life signs. The anesthesiologist, who normally could have helped a newcomer like me, had been called to another emergency, so I ended up working alone with a nurse who also had never been in a situation like this before. By Swami's grace, we were able to resuscitate the baby quickly. Everything was done in a routine manner, as if I had been used to doing this every day.

Another time, a nurse called me to look at a newborn baby. She said: "I really do not know what it is, but something is not quite right with this baby." "Sepsis," flashed through my head. This is a very serious bacterial infection in a newborn. I had learned to take these intuitive flashes seriously, even though in this case there was no maternal history to hint towards such a development nor were there any typical clinical signs. I drew blood, but the results came back negative. When I asked my colleague to look at the blood count again, she said: "Oh yes, you are right. This is a beginning sepsis." Of course, I knew that it was not me but Swami that made the correct diagnosis. The baby was transferred to a neonatal ward; treatment was started early enough, and all went well.

One night, I was on duty in the outpatient department. It was very busy. Amongst many other kids, there was a one and a half-year-old girl with her father. She was very difficult to examine, because she wouldn't stop screaming. Both she and her father did not speak a word of German or any other language I knew. Palpating her abdomen I, again, reacted very intuitively and called my colleagues from the children's surgical department telling them I suspected appendicitis. They were not very pleased and, in the beginning, did not want to look at her because, very often, they were consulted when somebody wanted to rid themselves of their responsibility. Also, appendicitis is rare at this age, and there were no laboratory findings yet. However, I persisted. Unfortunately, she was only operated on the following afternoon and, by that time, the appendix had already ruptured. However, in the end, all was okay.

Another experience where Swami took care of me was so unusual that it is worth telling even though it is only tangentially related to my medical practice. During my long stay at the ashram, in the summer of 1990, I had to go to Malaysia to get my visa renewed. Just before leaving, I was hoping that Swami would give a friend of mine permission to go with me but, instead, during darshan He said to me: "I will go with you!" Nobody else understood, but I heard Him clearly.

In Malaysia, a fellow Sai devotee was a perfect host and took care of me in such a loving way. When it was time to return, my flight back was in the middle of the night. I had always been scared of taking taxis at night, so I booked a car from the hotel to take me to the airport. The driver was especially nice and the whole atmosphere in the car so exceptionally warm and peaceful that I forgot my fear immediately and enjoyed the most extraordinary conversation.

"Which religion are you?" the driver asked me.

"I am a Christian."

"And I am a Muslim. You know, there are many similarities between Christianity and Islam."

"Well," I thought to myself, "I have doubts about that," but didn't say anything in order not to hurt his feelings. Until then, I had always had some prejudice against the Muslim religion, mainly because of the status women are given in most Muslim countries.

He then started to quote by chapter and verse from the *Bible* and the *Koran*, finding parallels between the two. This left me totally flabbergasted and also a bit ashamed, because this Malaysian taxi driver knew the *Bible* much better than I did. Then he asked:

"In the Gospel of John, Jesus said: "The one who sent me will come. Do you know who this is?"

It was as if a floodgate had opened. I started to tell Him all about Swami and could hardly stop talking. Later in the conversation, he asked me if I was working for the Indian government. He also said that it was such a pity that we didn't meet earlier, because we could have talked much more. When he dropped me at the airport, I was slightly surprised that this lovable gentleman didn't help me to take my luggage out of the trunk. However, at the time, I gave it no further thought.

When I told a friend of mine about my unusual taxi experience, she immediately exclaimed: "This was Swami!" "No, no," I replied, "quite impossible; he was a guy from the hotel; he was wearing the same shirt as they all did; and he has also given me his card."

Arriving at the ashram, I hurriedly dropped my luggage, quickly changed and rushed to darshan. I couldn't believe my eyes when I saw our little group being called for an interview. Standing at the door, Baba gave me a wonderful smile and said: *Less luggage, more comfort.* Still, I didn't understand. During the course of the interview when Swami spoke, He repeated the thoughts that I had when I was in Malaysia. "He really has been with me," I thought to myself.

Approximately half a year later, I had a sudden realization that Jesus had never said that the one who sent Him would come again. Only Swami had said this in one of His Christmas discourses. Jesus said that HE would come again! You can imagine how exited I was! I frantically started looking for this passage in the *Bible* but couldn't find it. The next morning, I went to the house of an Indian family to pick up a picture of Swami. I couldn't believe it but, above their door, there was a little wooden sign saying: I WILL COME AGAIN, the Gospel of John. There was no longer any doubt that this Malaysian taxi driver had been the Lord who, out of His boundless love, came to me in one of the many manifestations of His form. I was so awed. Knowing now that Swami Himself had been my charioteer, I tried to understand the Gita that He had given me.

I pondered over the questions the driver had asked me. Do I work for the Indian government? I looked at this symbolically. To me, India stands for spirituality and our way back home. In this way, the one who governs or rules this journey would obviously be the Lord Himself. Then the Lord's question to me would be: "Do you work for Me?" I believe He didn't expect me to answer right away but wanted to give me guidelines for my working life, as if to say: "Remember, nothing else matters out there. Do not be deceived; do not get entangled in running after name and fame! But work for Me, for My sake alone. Use this question as a tool to help you to practice constant self-inquiry. Do not tire in your efforts, strive for the purification of motives and aim at the total surrender of the fruits of action!"

The other casual remark the taxi driver had made was that it is a pity that we didn't meet earlier. This had deep significance to me, not only for my working life but life in general. Before I left Puttaparthi to go to Malaysia, I had met some of the "old-timers" who told wonderful stories of the golden times when there were only a handful of Westerners at the ashram and Swami came to visit them every day. They were allowed to cook for Him and to sleep in the mandir. One of the ladies even used Swami's footstool as her pillow! Seeing that Swami had become less and less available over the years, I used to lament: "Oh, Swami, it is such a pity that I didn't meet you earlier; we could have talked much more." When the Malaysian taxi driver said these exact same words to me, I gave him the following answer: "No, no, all is planned by God; everything is perfect the way it is." Swami had answered my plea through my own words! When we stop wanting things to be different from what they are, we can start to feel God's love and grace in every little detail of our life's journey. Then we can *live in the present,* as Swami says, *not ordinary presence, omnipresence!*

In the *Bhagavad Gita,* Sri Krishna teaches Arjuna the three steps to reach this divine love. He says: *"Work for Me! Work for my sake alone! Be devoted to Me!"* I strongly feel that this is what Swami was telling me to do.

These are only a few examples of Swami's unseen hand acting through me. Sometimes, He does this in a miraculous and spectacular way; sometimes, it is inconspicuous and seemingly accidental.

In all these cases, and in many other situations, prayer has been a constant companion and comforter. When I was doing my internship, I often assisted in open-heart surgery. During the procedure, the heart is cooled down for the protection of the heart muscle. I had to hold the heart in my hand without moving so that the anastomosis of the vessels, during the bypass operation, could be done properly. Very often, I was in a position where I could not even see the operation. Instead of feeling bored, I made it a practice to say the 108 names of God and prayed for the patient on the operating table. All the operations where I assisted were successful, and I hope that my prayers were able to make a small contribution.

I also had great joy in singing a special song of blessing to the newborn babies when they have their first physical examination. I always felt they need a warmer welcome than a doctor's stethoscope.

It is quite easy to praise the Lord as long as everything is going well. But how much more difficult is it to remain calm when our faith is put to the test? I remember once being falsely accused of having failed in a critical situation. There was nothing I could do to prove that I had not even treated that patient. *Fame and blame, just the same* was my lesson here. The only thing I could do was to surrender to the Lord. And there is such sweetness in doing so.

In medicine, as well as in every day life, I have one constant prayer, that Phyllis Krystal teaches, and which I feel is immensely powerful and wise. I ask Swami to think, feel, speak, act and love through me. The more I ask Swami to come into my life, the bigger the space He can adopt. The more I stand aside, the easier He can come through. The more I surrender, the smoother life flows. This is a process of eventually becoming as hollow as Krishna's flute.

Any process of lasting transformation is never rapid. It takes deep self-inquiry, work and practice. Many of my character weaknesses that I have been struggling with I am still struggling with now, being successful sometimes, and falling back into old habits at others. Still, the quality of the battle with ourselves changes; it is like on a spiral staircase, we come back to the same theme but on a different level. As I once heard a famous Austrian pediatrician say after a long scientific meeting, "I am still confused but on a higher level." Thus, I take consolation in one of Swami Yogananda's sayings, "A holy man is a sinner that never gave up." While we are in no way able to monitor our own progress and, perhaps, should not even attempt to do so, I do think that our path towards unity leads us through the field of compassion. Very often, we need to have our own painful experiences to soften our hearts to make us feel more deeply with our fellow man. For example, I think that having my own baby will greatly enhance my empathy for desperate, sleepless, and helpless parents. I will be able to feel more deeply with them and the screaming newborn when they storm the out patient department in the middle of the night.

Our sensitivity towards the needs and sufferings of our brothers and sisters will determine the depth of our commitment towards those who come to seek our help. I do believe that it is our responsibility to implement Swami's teaching when He says:

Duty without love is deplorable.
Duty with love is desirable.
Love without duty is divine.

Peace of Mind
Ram K. Setty, M.D.

At the very outset, I would like to dedicate this article to our beloved Lord Sri Sathya Sai. I have been asked to write an article about how spirituality has changed my practice of medicine. Simply put, spirituality has given me 'peace of mind.' Despite several personal disasters that struck me during the last few years, spirituality has saved me from much mental anguish.

Peace of Mind
Between 1995 and 1997, several major catastrophic events occurred. All of them pertain to my medical practice and, thereby, to my future. Each one of them, either individually or collectively, could have destroyed my practice and me. Many of my colleagues and foes alike wondered how I survived these hostile happenings. Spirituality was my only savior.

In 1978, I started a cardiology practice in a small town north of Santa Barbara, California. I was one of six cardiologists practicing in the city. With God's grace, I had built a successful practice in spite of intense competition. That successful practice was the result of my deep commitment to my patients. Unfortunately, it was tainted with evils such as ego, wealth and power. I was totally immersed in worldly objects, which I know now are purely physical, temporary, and external. I used to consider money and power as everything in life. I was intoxicated with it. Socializing and partying were routine. Pomp and show were obvious in everything I did. Because of this, I had no peace of mind.

In 1990, I turned to spirituality because of certain events that took place in my family. I gradually became an avid reader of Swami's books and totally immersed myself in spirituality. Now that I understand spirituality better, I am saddened with the way I handled past events. I had given so much importance to money, power and position in society. Within a few years, and by Swami's grace, I was able to understand the core principles of spirituality and was fascinated with the advaita philosophy which says: we are atma, not the body, mind or intellect; everything and everyone in the universe is atma. This is what Swami implies when He says, *unity in diversity.*

Swami has said, *Vaidyo Naaraayana Harih* (the doctor is divine), and *Sarve Bhavanthu Sukhinaha, Sarve Santhu Niraamayaah* (all should be happy and free from suffering). Being a physician, these statements have had a powerful effect on me. I have been fortunate enough to attend a few of Swami's discourses where He discussed health issues. In one of the discourses, Swami discussed in detail how a doctor first becomes a *good doctor* and, later, becomes a *God doctor*. These statements have solidified my faith in spirituality and changed my behavior completely. From being a purely worldly doctor, I have now become a spiritual doctor. I have taken the gigantic step from "I am the doer" to "I am an instrument." The priorities of money, position and prestige were changed to service and compassion. However, at no time was a patient's care in jeopardy. I always took very good care of my patients. The way in which Swami has turned my life completely around is a true miracle. Of course, that is what Swami does best!

Three major events happened to me during the years 1995 to 1997, and it was spirituality that helped me to cope with them.

First, in 1995, managed healthcare hit my town in full force. Being a specialist in medicine, in order to survive I had to depend on contracts in cardiology from managed care companies. Managed care is a new fad in health care in the United States. In this setting, patients are assigned to a primary care doctor who makes all the decisions for the patient. Specialists are contracted by the insurance companies. By the good old "divide and conquer" method, the insurance companies give a cheaper rate to the specialists. Also, in this type of healthcare, the patients have no direct access to see the specialist of their choice. The primary care doctor has certain restrictions placed on him by the insurance companies which pressure him to refrain from referring his patients to specialists. When a specialist is absolutely necessary, he can only refer to a contracted specialist who is with his own health plan. So, in this new game, specialists have little choice except to try and get contracts from the insurance companies. This was my predicament in 1995 when I was successfully edged out of all the contracts by my competition.

This stunned many of my colleagues and friends. Many predicted that my practice would be doomed, and I would leave the area within two to three years. But I was calm and confident. I did not bother with all of the commotion. I was continually praying to Swami and practicing spirituality. I knew these temporary and worldly things did not matter, and so I concentrated on the Permanent One. I left everything to Swami and surrendered to His lotus feet.

My patients appreciated my honesty, hard work and loving care. Gradually, by word of mouth, my practice attracted more new patients. I actually have more patients now than before when only doctors were referring new patients to me. There is no question in my mind who is behind this. I simply continued to do what I was doing before and lived a normal life. The peace of mind Swami gave me was like a shot of adrenaline. That gave me the confidence needed to keep the depressing situation well under control.

Then, in 1997, I had a major embezzlement in my office. A long time employee, who appeared to be trustworthy, virtually took me to the cleaners. By God's grace, I found out about the theft quickly; but by that time, I had lost close to a six figure amount of money. Every doctor in town, every nurse in the hospital, and every patient in my hometown, knew of the events which had occurred in my office. My competition started to circulate rumors that my practice was for sale and that I was leaving the area. But, once again, Swami took control of the situation by giving me tremendous strength and courage. I was able to see the situation as *passing clouds,* to quote Swami's words. I kept my equanimity in this turmoil, hoping the situation would change into a brighter day when the clouds would disappear. Without much fuss, I took out a huge loan, tightened my office expenses, cut my salary, and kept my office staff happy by not lowering their salaries. Over a period of time, my situation slowly improved. In mid 1998, I was able to pay off my debt and start earning my usual salary. Now, I am back to where I was before. Without my background in spirituality, I would have been in *pieces* instead of *peaceful*.

The third event that happened was in 1996 when a well-established and trustworthy office manager left me. She also took with her another key employee who was doing both nursing and transcribing. At this same time, I was having financial difficulties. Once again, I was not agitated at all, remembering Swami's teachings that *everything happens for good when one's intention is good*. Without any advertisement, a young woman came into my office seeking a position. She had little job experience and had no references, but my gut feeling told me otherwise. I hired her on the spot, and she proved to be far superior to my previous employee. It is very obvious to me who had sent her! I did not let these things bother me and can now see, from this experience, that the bad events turned out to be blessings in disguise.

As you can see, Swami has trained me well to withstand life's blows. I did not lose sleep. I did not lose my appetite. I did not see a psychiatrist. I did not resort to tranquilizers or sleeping pills. As a matter of fact, I slept fine during this turmoil. These events have made me strong, and my faith in spirituality has increased several fold. My love and respect for our beloved Lord Sai went sky high. His teachings on advaita helped me to conquer these difficult events more easily. This non-dualism theory is more valuable than all the money I have earned in this birth, and perhaps it is more valuable than the combined wealth of all my previous births. That is how much I owe to our dearest Lord Sai.

Injection of Love

Swami has taught us that love alone can conquer anything. It gives us tremendous power. It is more powerful than the atom bomb. This love is what is needed in medical practice. Doctors are in an excellent position to practice this love principle. Doctors can cure patients much better by talking to them with smiling faces, with sweet and soothing words, and by radiating love and compassion. Doctors are supposed to give courage and strength to ailing patients. A doctor should see the patient as his friend, interested in his health, not in the wealthy doctor's wallet. This is the key to a successful medical practice. This is what spirituality in medicine is all about. As Swami says, *Leave the animal qualities like ego, desire and anger behind and practice human qualities like love, compassion and sacrifice.* This is an ideal teaching for a physician to be successful in his or her practice.

Practice Before you Preach

A doctor should first practice spirituality before he applies it to his practice and teaches his patients. After all, spirituality means to know who you are. It is not just singing bhajans or sitting in meditation. Once you know that you are atma and everybody else is also atma, then you are practicing what Swami calls *unity in diversity.* This feeling will help doctors tremendously in their practice. Doctors can also, by virtue of their position, teach these principles of spirituality to their patients. This is best done not in words but by setting an example for the patient. When the patient sees how you lead your life, he will soon learn and incorporate the necessary changes in his own behavior. It will not be easy at first, but it can be done. I have certainly witnessed subtle changes in some of my hostile patients.

For example, Mr. J. A. came to see me for an initial visit a few months ago. His answers to all my questions were curt and filled with anger. I treated him the same way as I treat all my patients: with a loving voice, gentle reassuring touches, and showing a genuine interest in his health. Slowly, through a series of visits, he softened up. In fact, he actually referred three patients to me.

Prevention is Better than Cure

Doctors always talk about cure, but only a few concentrate on prevention. Even when they talk about prevention, they talk about it for the physical body. Swami has said that 80% of diseases arise from the mind. This is especially important to me as stress plays a major role in many diseases of the heart. If one looks beyond the present disease state, its onset and course, then one can see how the mind is responsible for the disease. The mind and its pollutants can be present in the patient for a long time before the onset of clinical symptoms. An interesting idea to contemplate is if the mind does not die until one is totally liberated, then perhaps disease states travel from birth to birth. Many things can pollute the mind, and food stands first. The mind is the key to health, so food must be carefully chosen so that it does not affect the mind.

Acceptance of the disease, the theory of karma and thinking of God are all important to consider. To teach these ideas to patients, especially in Western society, is very difficult. However, in a subtle way, with patience and persistence, a doctor can modify the lifestyle of his patients. One has to be very careful as he or she may be accused of being narrow minded and practicing voodoo or Eastern medicine. Our Lord Sai is always there to help us. One of the things I do when facing difficult patients is to keep humming a bhajan, loud enough for the patient to hear, and have a broad smiling face to go with it. Believe me, it works!

We Owe it to Society

It is very important to treat every patient the same way irrespective of cast, creed or economic status. Otherwise, it is a disaster for our spirituality. It is the doctor's duty to keep everyone healthy whether the patient pays or not. Recently, I saw a patient in the emergency room. He had no medical insurance and was cast off from one doctor to another. They treated his symptoms superficially, and not one of them did a complete work up. He had never had a follow up with any of the doctors. He was a sick man and needed aggressive management. Needless to say, I finally got him admitted to the hospital where his underlying problem was detected, and he was completely cured.

Swami has told us that society supports us, and we should show our gratitude by serving society. He has also suggested that doctors should serve at least one day a week in a free clinic, and that doctors should charge less for the people who cannot afford to pay. Alternatively, one can participate in free health clinics or fairs.

Spirituality has totally changed my life. Both my life and my practice are very peaceful. This peace of mind has given me the strength to face the difficulties of life with more ease. In difficult situations, remembering Swami's statement: *Everything is like passing clouds*, helps me. I have full faith in this, and this is what has kept me at peace. Also, the knowledge that difficulties bring you closer to God has helped me. With this newfound peace of mind, I am joyful in the office and happy in the hospital. Because I see everything I do as service, I can work long hours without feeling tired. Love and compassion are the primary tools in my practice. I am continually trying to implement Sai's teachings into my practice. Of course, I am far from achieving this. But, with His grace and blessings, one day I will make my practice an example of Sai spirituality.

You must have physical strength, spiritual strength and mental strength and, only when you have these three, can you really do service. Food, head and God: food is for the body, and you want a good body so the brain can function properly, so you can think. And why do you want this head and that intellect? To realize that which is beyond this – and that is God.

Sathya Sai Baba
Conversations with God, John Hislop, p 114

Swami is My Doctor
Rainer E. G. Ludwig, M.D.

Before I knew of Sathya Sai Baba and His teachings, I was a young family physician who was fairly stressed by the demands of a busy practice and a young family. It was my endeavor then to prevent illness, relieve suffering, and prevent death if at all possible. Office consultations, deliveries of babies, and house calls occupied much of my time, so that I left the raising of our two daughters primarily to my wife. Unbeknownst to me at the time, my wife increasingly felt alone. In her distress, she made demands of a material nature, wanting a bigger house and more spending money which, of course, required more work on my part outside the house. We both felt stressed and misunderstood and slipped into an accusatory style of communication.

Unconsciously, I began to feel more comfortable outside of our home and, therefore, spent even more time away. During that period, the young wife of one of our best friends was diagnosed with a terminal illness. Big questions arose for which there were no immediate answers. Is there life after death? Where do we go after this life on earth is finished? What is the purpose of life? Our friend was able to take time off from work and stay home to look after his wife. He read many authoritative books on these topics. Whatever literary gems he came across, he would give me to read. The first book that made a deep impression on me was *Autobiography of a Yogi* by Paramahansa Yogananda. The next book led me to read late into the night; I would often catch myself holding my breath while discovering the deep truths described by Dr. Samuel Sandweiss in *Sai Baba, The Holy Man and the Psychiatrist.* Halfway through this book, tears came to my eyes, tears of immense relief. This happened to me – a man who had not shed a tear since childhood, and to eyes that one of my preceptors in medical training had described as icy-cold, like steel. I was so relieved and excited about this great teacher by the name of Sai Baba that I was determined to see Him one day. I decided to check into the validity of the contents of books on this teacher of teachers, and on His leelas, after preparing myself by becoming a vegetarian, avoiding alcohol, and reading more about this holy man.

Gradually, I expanded my outlook on life from one based on Western philosophy to the broader, Eastern point of view, which sees human life as a continuum rather than an isolated, finite event. I visited Swami in India and observed Him. Through His person, I became convinced that there was a God, and that God was easily recognizable in the form of this holy man. I became aware that the Bible and its accounts of the life of Jesus could also very well be true. Thus, I turned from an agnostic viewpoint to one that accepted that God was everywhere. Our office staff recalls that on my return from visiting Baba there was a glow about me. I was happy to share what I had read and experienced with anyone, and even sometimes when it wasn't asked for!

I had Swami on my mind constantly, and made a mental game out of looking for him inside patient's ears and throats. Whatever I did for a patient, such as clipping the thickened toenails of an elderly patient, I pretended to do it for Swami. Whenever difficulties would arise, I would silently address Swami inside and say, "Swami, I don't know what is going on here. What should be done? Please see through me, think through me, and speak through me." Invariably, peace would come to my racing mind. Frequently, whatever happened next would resolve the dilemma.

One such memorable instance occurred when I was on call and received an early morning phone call from a concerned mother who was always a very reliable observer and never bothered with trivial things. It was the middle of the influenza season, and one of her children was taken ill. We decided that I would make a detour to visit the child at home before going to the office. Both parents and two other siblings were eagerly awaiting my diagnosis. I reviewed the history, examined the patient, and leaned toward the impression that the likeliest diagnosis was, indeed, influenza. As I started to explain my reasons for this diagnosis to the girl and her parents, I also realized that I was not very sure of my diagnosis concerning the vague and "soft" abdominal findings. Silently, I asked Swami to take over. As I was preparing to leave, I looked back over my shoulder at the young patient who was at that very moment grimacing as she tried to sit up in bed. She affirmed that her lower abdomen had hurt as she was changing positions. I quickly changed my presumptive diagnosis and sent her to Children's Hospital where, later that day, the pediatric surgeon took out an appendix that was about to burst.

Much later, the astute mother asked me what had changed my mind that morning with respect to her daughter's illness at a time when many people suffered from abdominal cramping, nausea, and vomiting. I admitted then that I had not been sure but had guessed at the diagnosis of flu on the basis of a greater probability. Feeling uneasy about that assumption, I had asked inwardly to be shown the truth, or for God to work through me. I do not know how I came to look back at the patient just as she made a face on sitting up. However, I do recall feeling relieved after I made the less probable diagnosis of appendicitis as the likeliest cause of our young patient's discomfort. Once that diagnosis proved correct during surgery, I was astonished to feel a certain sense of pride at having made the right decision, even though I knew that I had had a lot of help that day. I knew that the feeling of pride was misplaced and should have been replaced by a deeper sense of gratitude.

Meanwhile, the situation at home continued to deteriorate. My attendance at a local Sai center, where many pictures and statues of strange figures, as well as songs frequently sung in a foreign language, did little to relieve the concerns amongst my family members and neighbors who thought I had fallen in with a cult. Through the help of friends, a psychiatrist was contacted in order to try and help resolve the rift between my wife and myself. He announced one day that he saw me as an angry man. "I am not angry!" I almost shouted. Inwardly, I said to myself, "How can I possibly be angry when Swami refers to us as embodiments of love!" It was only much later that I realized the lack of self-analysis on my part. I had suppressed and ignored feelings and relied almost solely on ideas and my mind to get me through life. The sense of duty and preoccupation with learning and applying skills in medicine had not included an honest inner appraisal of feelings and emotions, which lie closer to our innermost being than mental gymnastics. Our capable psychiatrist suddenly died and left us struggling with unresolved issues. Another counselor gave up all hope of salvaging the marriage after only three sessions. Instead of going through more explorations for the reasons of the failing marriage, I retreated into studying Swami's books, meditation, and attending more meetings at the Sai center where the vibrations were always positive.

While we lived in this state of cohabitation, I visited Swami once more in Puttaparthi. As providence would have it, someone called me to help a couple from Australia. The wife had busied herself in all kinds of service opportunities outside of her home where she felt appreciated and valued. On the other hand, her older husband had increasingly felt more isolated and rejected. As a result, he had withdrawn into himself, becoming depressed and suicidal. His point of view was that his wife's priority in service should be to dedicate herself to looking after his needs. I listened to both of them and, then, suggested how they could deal with the problem by trying to resolve the impasse at home first, rather than putting so much effort into outside activities. Clearly, Swami was forcing me to look at my own situation by presenting me with an identical problem in another marriage. Even so, I did not take my own advice. Instead of following Swami's teachings of "doing first, then telling," I told only, and neglected my advice with my own family. In other words, I followed the path of least discomfort and tried not to get into any arguments. My wife did not know Swami's teachings, but she was afraid of poverty and the derision from neighbors should I decide to give up all our material wealth to what she called "that cult." Eventually, lawyers were engaged, and I was advised to move out of the house.

Through the process of estrangement, separation, and divorce, I kept my mind on Swami, His wonderful leelas, and His teachings. Even though there were, indeed, difficult times while I was still in the house and while preparing for divorce later on, I never once had difficulty sleeping or felt agitated when I was alone. After I had moved into an apartment, a neighbor walked up to me in the grocery store to exchange greetings. As she approached me, she suddenly threw up her arms in great astonishment exclaiming, "What peace is around you!" I was indeed thankful to Swami for granting me health and an honorable profession, even though I had failed miserably at marriage. Resignation to what I saw as His will made me gladly accept anything as long as I felt He was with me.

While practicing bringing Swami's presence into my daily life, I would put a little food on a plate for Him. Doubting the sanity of such actions, I spoke to Swami in my mind. "How is it, Swami, that You appear to others in the physical world, but You never even eat a little bit of what I put out for You?" Without further thought, I put a wrapped candy on His plate on the dining room table and prepared to do the dishes. Suddenly, the curtain moved, and a squirrel came from the ground floor balcony into the dining room. It hopped around the table, onto the chair next to the plate and, from there, onto the tabletop. The squirrel picked up the candy with its front paws and peeled off the wrapper with its teeth. Within seconds, the animal retreated with the candy back out to the balcony leaving me holding my breath in disbelief at what had just happened. Has Swami not said that all names and forms are His?

Despite this hint of His omnipresence, I kept looking at Swami as the giver of boons and the embodiment of truth who would give me the key of how to disentangle myself from the vagaries of the mind and find God. And so it happened that He gave me first row for darshan in Puttaparthi. On this particular occasion, my mind was unusually clear. Before the Lord came, I had a premonition as to where He would walk, where He would stop to take letters and, that if He stopped in a particular square of slate flooring in front of me, it would be a sign to take the hoped-for padnamaskar. When Swami entered the Sai Kulwant Hall minutes later, He walked just as in a replay on TV. He stopped in the precise square and looked at me. Instinctively, I rested my forehead on His soft feet, sat back, and looked up at Him. I was confused since there was no particular joy or elation following this activity. All I noticed was that Swami was looking expectantly, like a mirror, back at me. I was left unfulfilled and empty as Swami continued giving darshan.

After some rumination, I came to the conclusion that Swami wanted me to look inside rather than at His physical form to find the answers to the riddles of life and self-realization. He started me on this path by giving me a friend who had been practicing self-inquiry for a long time and who insisted, through questioning me, that I check to see how I feel. Now feelings were things I had been trying to ignore for most of my life. By inquiry, I learned that feelings are closer to the truth I was seeking than mental explorations, which tend to spring from ego and are quite often the opposite of spiritual truth. Getting into the habit of naming the feeling gave rise to other questions of how these feelings came about. In this way, I discovered how I had colored events in my early life with the brush of fear of inadequacy. Once this happened, any subsequent reaction or response was, thereafter, made from the perception that I had been offended. The reaction usually came in the form of a sarcastic comment or a criticism. By practicing becoming the observer of the mind, I am now learning to let go of negative responses and react spontaneously in loving kindness, which is closer to who I really am.

Swamiji, in His compassion, had already given me an earlier experience that should have torn away the veil of ignorance. It was during a ceremony when Swami inaugurated the grounds where the Super Specialty Hospital was to be built. Swami had arranged for various dignitaries and doctors, who had served during the birthday celebrations in the medical camp, to be assembled under tents on that radiant morning. Swamiji most graciously introduced those who were involved in the project. He did this with unequaled charm pointing out in a most loving way how the various dignitaries had excelled in their duties. Then, He stopped talking and walked past the doctors blessing everyone with His upturned palm circling in the air. All our eyes were riveted on Swami. All thought ceased, and an overwhelming, intense, joyful energy seemed to be both within and around me. I hardly dared breathe or move, much less speak, so full of awe was I in observing this wonderful feeling of love and bliss that the Lord had brought forth. As I write and recollect these events, it becomes clear to me that we are that love energy I experienced that day. So, Swamiji's message is that we should practice recognizing the same indweller in everyone by abandoning the mental habit of judging and developing love instead.

Despite these experiences, I do get into a panic when difficulties arise, and I forget God. Again, Swami showed that He was with me when I really needed Him. It began when a patient consulted me with respect to avoiding illness during her travels to Africa. We discussed the methods of malaria prevention that were available at the time, and which are still inadequate now. Unfortunately, she developed cerebral malaria weeks after her return from that continent and was near death as the illness evolved. She required both specialized acute care and months of rehabilitation before she was able to return to her prior employment. Her lawyer alleged that the medical advice I had given was negligent.

With Swami's divine guidance, a couple of unexpected events eased the stress of the litigation process. Firstly, the editor of the Canadian Sathya Sai Newsletter had asked me to write a travel advisory for people traveling to Puttaparthi. I had researched the subject matter, including the advice and methods for preventing malaria, and had written about it in an article of the newsletter that was published just prior to my patient's office visit. Hence, I could argue and prove that I was up-to-date regarding the subject matter at the time of her visit.

The next major help arrived in a fashion that was similarly comforting. As part of my defense, I had to contact the malpractice insurance company in order to obtain legal representation. The difficulty arose when I could not find my membership card. I knew that it was the size of a credit card and was somewhere in my possession. Every free moment I was looking for the card. I thought it would be in a particular drawer where I put most of the smaller items that I might need someday. I had already searched that drawer twice. Finally, I took the drawer out of its cabinet and emptied the contents onto the dining-room table. I also checked the sides and bottom of the drawer as well as the cabinet. Carefully, I replaced all the items into the drawer and thought, dejectedly, "Swami, I cannot find this membership card. I don't know where it is. If I am to have it, you'll have to help me!" I then gave up looking. As I prepared to leave the apartment moments later, I opened that same drawer. As I pulled it open, I saw something flutter face down onto the floor. Wondering, hoping, and almost knowing what it was, I bent down and turned over the card. It was the long–sought-after item! From that moment on, I had the deep conviction that Swami was involved in this ordeal. Relieved, I decided that my duty was to tell the truth to the best of my ability – whatever interpretation the legal system reached was beyond my control or influence. What comfort to know that Swamiji is the doer; it removed the role of victim and substituted the role of observer in its place! By His grace, the affair was settled out of court without attaching blame. Even years later, I feel no particular anger or frustration concerning this experience, but just relief that comes from applying Swami's teachings. Here are those teachings stated in their most exalted form:

He who appears to be nowhere, He is everywhere.

He who appears to be disinterested, He is enjoying everything.

He who appears to be doing nothing, He is doing everything.

All of the struggles of daily life cease once we appreciate that the same energy animates all of us. At the very core of our being, no one is better or worse than anyone else, because we are all one and the same. Where is the need for me to feel elated or to judge myself as superior when I have a pleasant experience? Conversely, it is only a mental projection when I feel offended or judge myself as inadequate or bad when a negative event takes place. We are not the experience.

We all prefer truth rather than lies, love rather than fear, justice rather than injustice, and peace rather than war. When we choose to act and respond with love and understanding along the lines of right conduct or goodness, our conscience is satisfied, inner struggles cease, and peace is established. However, the mind, with its worries and doubts, tends to create wants driven by fear of inadequacy. Swami advises us to "end the mind" so we can be our true selves.

Sometimes words just pour out of my mouth, which come from insights and the application of Swami's teachings in daily life. One such event occurred with the arrival of a new patient who had been referred by the family of the girl who had the appendectomy. This new patient was a judge who had been accused of manslaughter and was awaiting trial. Although obviously a bright middle-aged man, he felt quite guilty and depressed and suffered from insomnia. He related to me how, on a wet and overcast day, he was driving his sports car to the courthouse when a drunken man stepped off the curb into the path of his vehicle. That man had died as a result of injuries sustained in the mishap. The judge bemoaned the death of this unintentional victim and, in deep remorse, declared that, just because of his actions, the man who had died in the accident would never see the beauty of nature again. "How do you know that?" was my challenge. We quickly reviewed the question of who we are and disposed of the idea that we are the human body, which is constantly changing. Similarly, we concluded that we are not the mind either, which is nothing more than desires that frequently vary. We decided that we are the energy that makes us different from corpses. And, according to the laws of physics, as energy we are neither created nor destroyed, but carry on indefinitely. With respect to feeling guilty, he appreciated that such an interpretation was only appropriate if his actions were inconsiderate, wrong, or designed to create harm. My new patient did agree that it was, therefore, not necessary to feel the way he did. On a later occasion, he revealed that those insights had helped him a lot. After the court had ruled him innocent of any alleged misdeed he, of course, felt even more vindicated.

I find myself sharing some aspect of Swami's teachings on an almost daily basis with the patients He sends to me. In fact, Swami is the inner resident in these people who happen to be burdened by some fear or mental agitation. Just the other evening, a pre-teen boy asked me, while his parents were standing next to him, "Doc, what can you give me so that I grow big?" "What way do you want to be big?" I asked. "Do you want to be tall like a basketball player, or do you want to be great as a person like Mother Teresa? If you want to become exceptional, you have to develop character. I know you can do it! I've heard you sing a Shiva bhajan with tremendous energy even though your body is still not fully-grown. Learn to trust truth and the other human values as your guide in life. Follow and practice Swami's teachings and your life will be great!"

At special opportunities like these, there is no contemplation or thinking. The words just pour out of my mouth and joy, contentment, and love shine on the faces of all around, just like I see on the faces of the devotees during darshan time. Even though Swami's teachings are on my mind daily, and even though Swami tells us that He is always with us, I still have the urge to visit Him in the physical form whenever an opportunity presents itself. Each visit with the Master is different and not predictable. When a reliable substitute physician suddenly became available in November 1998, I hurried back to Puttaparthi once more. On most of my prior trips, Swami had spoiled me with beautiful darshans and even the occasional smile. During this latest visit, no matter how I tried, I could not get physically close to Him.

Quite by accident, I decided to go to the general hospital just as a meeting for the doctors who wanted to work in the medical camp was in progress. During the ensuing free medical clinics, the doctors from outside India were allowed to attend to the local population for the first time. During the next several days, we worked with a team of administrators, translators, paramedical and medical personnel in shifts around the clock. We were presented with a whole spectrum of diseases in very advanced stages. Chronic anemia due to parasites, advanced valvular diseases from rheumatic fever, tuberculosis in many unusual anatomical places were some of the illnesses that I had not seen before in clinical practice. There was often very little we could do, but I hope that by listening to the patient's complaints, at least we were showing compassion and sharing some of their burdens.

One man in particular stands out in my memory. Through an interpreter, he complained of chest pain. With his shirt removed, I was aghast at several foot-long and one inch-wide scars that crisscrossed his chest. Upon inquiring, I learned that these were the scars from a beating he had sustained years ago when villagers had attacked him with bamboo sticks. I wanted to know why he looked so skinny and sad. The man began to cry and answered in an unfamiliar language. The translator reported that our patient was worried about not being able to feed his seven children. He explained further that he used to provide for them by driving a truck but had not been able to drive because of failing eyesight. Two meals had been the sum total of what he had to eat in the last eight days! I learned that the only welfare system in India is a begging bowl. It is true that a deliberate government policy keeps the costs of medications at a low level; however, they are still out of reach for the poor. I trust that this man has had his cataracts removed at the Super Specialty Hospital by now.

What great opportunities we have as doctors to help the disadvantaged! Of course, it is the very poor who give the medical staff the opportunity to develop an altruistic attitude. They are the real devotees of Swami – they bear poverty and illness, that we could not tolerate, with such gracious equanimity that is beyond our understanding. It is my resolve to never judge slow-moving villagers again, for they might be in the end-stages of congestive heart failure. What reason do I have to complain, the foreigner who enjoys health and luxury, just because there is no seat for me inside the Sai Kulwant Hall during the Lord's birthday celebration? Should I not concentrate only on purifying my heart to make it an appropriate residence for God?

I am indebted to Swami in so many ways. First, I thank Him for giving me the opportunity to lead a noble life by letting me work as a physician. Next, I feel He has helped me when my personal life was at its deepest low by granting me peace without measure. By Swami's grace, my previously estranged children, who felt abandoned by me and unloved by their mother, have escaped disaster and are thriving young adults now. Through patience, the practice of listening and validating each other's point of view, a caring relationship has re-emerged between us! He continues to inspire and to strengthen my faith in altruistic principles through His own example and the authority of His teachings, which come from Truth.

Whenever difficulties arise, I shift my focus to Swami's name, or one of His leelas or teachings and, then, a joyful peace emerges, which enriches my daily life immensely. He is my idol, my strength, my God! He is goodness personified; He is my inner motivator; He is my conscience; He is the energy that gives life to my body and mind; He is my **All**. Without Him, I am naught. How can I thank Him except by following His teachings? He wants nothing back from us except the love that comes from Him and passes through us back to Him.

Thank you, Swami, for allowing me to become aware of Your presence and Your life, which is Your message! Without these, my life would be a depressing wasteland – unthinkable! Thank you for making us aware of greatness, beauty, and goodness. Through Your untiring efforts, You are making us aware of greater altruistic choices in our lives for the elevation of mankind. As I gradually follow Your example, I become aware of a transformation that is taking place within me. I am changing from a timid, reserved, and even cold person, to one who is more spontaneous, joyful, and caring. Encouraged by a sense of freedom associated with following Your teachings, whenever I am aware of a choice to be made, I now consciously select a path or response based on truth, understanding, and loving kindness.

Thinking of Swami as the energy of love that flows through me to His various forms has improved the doctor-patient relationship so much that I cannot now conceive of a life without Swami. It is really Swami's love and words of wisdom that the patients are receiving when I speak without ego. At those times, I also feel quite energetic and often hear advice suggesting alternatives nobler than those I would have thought of myself. Those options would no doubt improve the message of my own life if I were to practice them more consistently.

It behooves us all to recall the words of Mark Twain, the American humorist, who observed that, "Mother Nature heals and the doctor sends the bill!" Was he not suggesting that doctors are deluding themselves by taking credit for the healing process? To become wise and free from that delusion, we must establish the habit of following our inner motivator, our conscience, in carrying out our duty to the best of our ability and, through the practice of human values, recognize that God is the love energy that sustains us all. None of us is greater than the other; in fact, there is only One!

The Healing of the Doctor
Ricardo Gutierrez, M.D.

Since my childhood, there has been a family bias in favor of my attending medical school. My grandmother had stated that she would enjoy seeing me as a doctor, and my parents mentioned how proud they would feel if I became a physician. Family pressure was obviously carrying me in a definite direction. However, I was quite confused when I was sixteen, and it was the time to make this decision.

The deciding factor, however, was that I had made a promise to God—an unusual event that happened one day when I was in the last year of high school. My brother at the time was less than two years old. While playing in the backyard, he accidentally spilled a cup of kerosene over his face and, stunned, inhaled a bit of it. He immediately developed respiratory distress and very heavy coughing. While my parents tried to help him, he became red and blue in the face. I was really afraid that he would die. I knew from the movies that inhalation and ingestion of fuel by swimmers from sunken ships is usually fatal, and one of my school mates had died some months earlier from pneumonitis due to accidental inhalation of diesel oil.

I retreated into the house, all the while hearing the coughing of my brother and the shouting of my parents. I talked to God saying that if He permitted my brother to live, I promised to study medicine. I do not know the reason for this behavior of mine, because I was not on a religious path at the time, so believing I could entice God by studying medicine was really odd. My brother survived and, the fact is, I felt obliged by this promise, and this put an end to my ambivalence regarding the selection of a career.

For my family, medicine had the attraction of prestige and wealth. Not surprisingly, this was a significant factor in my own decision-making. In Argentina in 1963, there was no social security; the hospital was for the needy, and everyone else just paid cash. Doctors were the most conspicuously rich people in town.

When I recall my years at medical school, I see a mass of haphazard events only loosely bound together by student establishment and university rules. I felt as if I was dragging myself through time and study by mere inertia, governed by patches of concepts such as an obligation towards my parents, material convenience, and fear of whatever could happen if I did anything unusual.

It was during my stay as an intern that I eventually chose the pediatric residency. This choice mostly came from the impression collected during the last year at medical school, when a team of very caring and dedicated people taught the subject. I suspect I sensed a sort of tenderness in the pediatric environment, perhaps something that came from the whole endeavor of rearing children. One thing is certain, I was not a baby-lover type; as a pediatrician, I was shy and fearful, with little capability for heart-to-heart contact.

The all-pervading feeling of the uselessness of my life and the burden of my job plagued my early years. Many popular tangos in Argentina lend talented poetry to this complaint. "Ya sé, no me digás, tenés razón: la vida es una herida absurda," they sing. This means, "I know, don't say anything, you're right: life is just an absurd wound." Even when I started to work as a doctor, this feeling continued but, somehow, I managed to make an effort to do things well for the patients.

My healing began to take place before the advent of Swami into my consciousness. About eleven years ago, I became interested in the Indian sage, Sri Ramana Maharshi, then the *Bhagavad Gita*, which for a time became my bedside book. But finally, I came to feel that I did not need to part from my Catholic history and environment. Any religion would do for the purpose of approaching God. So I turned my attention to Catholic doctrine and the Western saints, reading about the mystical experiences of San Juan de la Cruz and Santa Teresa de Avila.

Teilhard de Chardin is another link that brought me to Baba. He acted as a bridge for me to join science with faith. Before I knew Swami, Teilhard's writings helped me add to my work some of the sweetness coming from God in the form of Jesus. Pierre Teilhard de Chardin played the important role of bringing the two worlds together. A renowned paleontologist and a philosopher, he was also a Catholic priest. A fervent evolutionist, he envisioned creation as a continuum, progressing from the shapeless, as it emerges from God, to the shaping of the Universe, on to the creation of life, humans and finally, to the arrival of mankind back to God. The bridging from reason to faith was crucial for me, as I was one who was afflicted by the illusion that puts mind and its conceptions above all else.

It was a long process for me to become a devotee of Sri Sathya Sai Baba. For about two years, a friend of mine gently prodded me along. It began with a book on yoga that went beyond body postures, describing a way in which man could rendezvous with God. Next I read *Autobiography of a Yogi* by Swami Yogananda. Then, by my own initiative, came Arthur Osborne's book on Sri Ramana Maharshi and several other works on Ramana's teachings. The first book directly mentioning Swami was *Sai Baba, the Holy Man and the Psychiatrist* by Dr. Samuel Sandweiss. It was strange how I discovered I was a devotee. This friend, having moved to another province, returned after several months for a brief visit. His first question to me was, "So, do you believe in Baba now?" I carefully looked inside myself for a moment and then said, "Yes."

In 1997, when I became a devotee, I was fortunate to stumble upon words of Swami saying that whatever happens, whatever is experienced, is His will. Of all the teachings I received from my family, the one I am the most thankful for is the crucial concept of eternity. This was a gift given to me at an early age by my grandmother so that it could stay embedded in my mind. She made me understand that, after death, we can be with God forever and ever and ever... I believe the concepts we feel most comfortable with are usually the ones that arise by default when under pressure; they are the ones given to us during the very assembling of our minds.

This concept of eternity enabled me to exercise some discrimination, not in a conscious way, but as the underlying reason for my feeling that I do not fit into the material world. For years, I had the vague sensation of discomfort about worldly life. I felt that "this" could not be what it is all about. I was inadvertently discriminating between what is false and true, sensing that all this was false. I believe this was the driving force that pushed me to be a seeker.

This past year, I have been experimenting with healing two of my own illnesses by the use of vibhuti. One is chronic sinusitis, the other arthrosis of the cervical spine. Both of these began ten years ago.

During this period, I was on and off of antibiotics for the sinusitis, and have undergone surgery to tap my maxillary sinuses. Relapses of sinusitis are announced by a state of malaise, severe chills, face pain, and purulent nasal discharge soon follows. In order to treat my sinusitis, I started to inhale vibhuti through my nostrils twice a day. Although I had never heard or read about inhaling vibhuti this way, I felt confident that nothing would go wrong since everything comes from Baba. After a few days, the usual relapse did not show up. I have not had any antibiotics whatsoever for the last year. Although I have had several colds during this period, instead of the expected sinus complications, nothing happened, and the colds smoothly went away.

The other ailment that I treated successfully with vibhuti was cervical arthrosis. This began without warning with a pain in the back of my neck at the base of my head. I have had to wear a collar as well as take anti-inflammatory medication once or twice a day. It took me six months to stop using the collar, by which time I became addicted to the anti-inflammatory pills, which masked the symptoms and resulted in a need for another pill to treat gastritis.

I was already free of the need for sinus medication when another friend of mine complained about his stuffed nose, a nuisance he endured for years. He resorted to steroid injections with increasing frequency. My friend was not aware that, among other things, steroids have the attendant side effects of immunodepression and osteoporosis. Sensing my disapproval of this therapeutic approach, he asked me to treat him. I, at once, thought of prescribing him vibhuti.

Coincidentally, I had just been reading a story about Mahatma Gandhi where a lady begged him to tell her son to withdraw from adding salt to meals, since the doctors had told him he must do so. Gandhi told them to come back two weeks later. On the second visit, he kindly used all the weight of his prestige to formally counsel the boy. The woman then asked why Gandhi did not speak to him in the first interview. The answer was that, before feeling he was able to prescribe to someone else, he had to quit salt himself, which he had done during the two previous weeks.

I was impressed by this conduct, so I decided that I must first quit the pain pills that I had been taking for ten years, and I began to use the vibhuti instead. Twice daily, I would swallow a little and use another bit to massage the base of my skull and back of my neck. As expected, pain appeared the next day, but this time things were different. I was somehow more detached from my body. I could take the pain without so much anguish, or the sensation of impending doom that pain brings with it. Very gradually, over a period of days, the pain subsided. I was really happy. Ten days after my last pill, I arranged to see my friend, telling him I was going to treat him with a new recipe: vibhuti. He started nose inhalations at once. My friend has experienced an overall improvement; nevertheless, in the beginning of the treatment, he had a temporary relapse which forced him to resort, only once, to his well-known steroid shot. He occasionally feels some nasal congestion, but as he persists in using vibhuti, there is steady improvement. This is in spite of his noncompliance with regular allergy prescriptions, such as avoiding cats and restricting his diet. He has now quit the nasal applications and is only taking vibhuti orally.

A third healing that took place with vibhuti was the healing of my migraines. Migraines are periodic headaches accompanied by nausea or vomiting and a state of general discomfort. I consider this a real boon, because I didn't intentionally seek this as I did with my other two conditions.

This condition has plagued me consistently from the age of thirty, though I recall isolated attacks that began when I was in elementary school. After coming to Baba, I quit migraine drug treatment altogether. Now, when I feel the initial stages of a migraine, I take vibhuti orally and massage it over the tender area on my head. Usually, relief occurs within one hour. There have been occasions when the pain did not totally subside. However, the severity of the bouts is much less than it used to be. I must state that, nowadays, the frequency of relapses is very low.

I would like to tell one more tale on the efficacy of vibhuti. During the meeting of the regional branch of the Sathya Sai Organization, I was exhausted from traveling by bus all night. The fatigue, coupled with some anxiety at attending such a special occasion, prompted the well-known head and neck pain that I have come to identify in its early stages. I immediately took vibhuti, swallowing a bit and massaging another portion over my neck and head. In a matter of half an hour, the pain was gone.

For a year, I have not had any medication. There are occasional spells of neck pain in stressful situations or physical strain, but they subside in a day or two with a regimen of several doses of vibhuti per day, orally and massaged. Nevertheless, I am in a dilemma. On the one hand, I have the desire to leave everything in His hands. Yet, He advises us that our effort is essential. Does the effort mean that a physician, who is a devotee of Swami, should use all the available medical weaponry to treat his own diseases? After a lot of thought about this, I have come to feel that, perhaps, the vibhuti will not always bring about a physical cure; but what matters most to me now is the spiritual change. And this means turning my confidence toward God instead of medication.

Although I had begun to change during the period when I concentrated on the Catholic approach, becoming a Sai devotee has accelerated this process. There have been substantial shifts in my overall behavior and personality. I have quit smoking, drinking alcoholic beverages, and have become a vegetarian. I can honestly say I am a better doctor than before. I used to have a technical approach towards medicine. I saw myself as the administrator of a certain amount of useful information, and I dispensed it in a cold, mechanical way.

Barking prescriptions to patients is something Baba would specifically discourage. When I occasionally find myself slipping into this behavior, I remember His words to cool down, and I take this as a reminder of where I really am on the spiritual path. Nevertheless, I can say I enjoy a better rapport and a warmer relationship with patients.

I have even begun to receive some spontaneous recognition from patients and parents. Kids have shown pleasure in coming to my office, as their Dad or Mom would jokingly comment.

Before Swami and my involvement with spirituality, when I examined children, I would stare at them, use the sthetoscope, tongue depressor, othoscope, weigh and measure them, all as if I were manipulating pieces of machinery. I had the habit of doing the near minimum for my patients. I would listen to the reasons for the visit and devote only the time strictly needed for the problem. Currently, I pay attention to items beyond the obvious consult, namely: family affairs which may influence the outcome, assorted achievements of the child, immunizations, which in my environment is partially subject to the initiative of the attending physician, and nutrition and supplementation, which are defective as a rule in segments of our population. Obviously, these are regular items that any good pediatrician would take care of. In my case, it is clear that Swami has been the one responsible for the "healing of the doctor."

Nowadays, children frequently bother their parents in the waiting room trying to get in before the assigned schedule so they can play and/or eat candies. In my office, I have a riding car, a rugged inflatable riding horse, a set of big assembling pieces, soft piling cubes, a ball, a big box, and a tray of candies. There are also framed paintings by children on the wall. Often, a child comes in crying with fear. But when it is time to leave, he or she has to be, literally, dragged out by the mother.

What I previously considered superfluous, I am now doing: playing and chatting with the kids and talking with the parents. I have even found myself hugging children or taking babies in my arms. Because of all these changes, I like to think there has been a "divinization" of my practice. As I have had a more human attitude, the overall outcome of my patients has also improved.

I believe now that I am His instrument and, therefore, I must be a good one. I must put whatever free will He has given me to steadily move towards the values He promotes: Love, Truth,

Peace, Righteousness and Non-violence. Using these guidelines, I try to weigh my choices carefully. Clearly, it is I who will ultimately benefit from this effort.

I know I have lots of work to do. I can still become anxious for the queue of patients to come to an end so that I can leave the office. Or, sometimes, I feel bored with repeating the set of prescriptions for common cold or basic nutrition. Unfortunately, every now and then, I catch myself in a fit of the olden-day ignorance, losing my temper with some parent, nurse, or colleague. I feel ashamed to recall how boldly I showed these traits during my first years of practice.

However, I am trying to see Swami's hand in everything and remember Him during work, particularly when I am about to make a difficult decision. Remembering Him means that I am telling Him, "Let Your will prevail." I try to remember that, whatever happens, it is His will, and I will accept the outcome of this action be it good or bad to my limited understanding. All these thoughts are packed within the name "Om Sai Ram," or "Swami," or in a flash of His image. I try to remember that all who enter the consulting room are incarnations of God, Swami in disguise.

Another aspect of my behavior prior to Swami, which is only tangential to medicine, concerns my confusion about money, its management, earning, administration, use or misuse. I have been profoundly ignorant on the subject of wealth. I even used to feel satisfaction at this handicap of mine, wrongly identifying it as detachment from material possessions. Therefore, I felt no guilt for my faults in this area: spending more than I earned, and problems with my bank account due to mistakes in my checkbook. In order to preserve my dear ego, I saw things upside-down, deeming virtuous what is really a defect! I realize, now, I was just oblivious to my own ignorance and laziness. With Swami's help, I now understand that correct action encompasses proper management of money, and that wealth, having no intrinsic evil, can be used for good or bad purposes.

Something I could never have done prior to Swami is to take care of my father in the way I am doing now. When he first came to live with me, I saw his presence as a hindrance to my style of life. Now, I give Dad top priority. I do not plan any schedule that would prevent my accompanying him daily for breakfast and lunch—he has supper with the maid during my evening office hours. I spend weekends with him and cook for him. Occasionally, I accompany him to pay a visit to my brother who lives in the same town and, in the night, we come back early as he likes. Before, I used to stay late for conversation, oblivious of my father's muffled scorn.

Daily routine is a bit of a test, as my father forgets what he has just said or done. He is afflicted by senile amnesia with some degree of cognitive impairment. I am sad about him because, at eighty-four years, he is aware of his limited life span. This gives him a mixture of fear and anger with no way to soothe the pain. Chatting consists, on his part, in repeating endlessly some simple observation, for instance about the weather—with the best of intentions of making good conversation. The tactic is, of course, to always answer as kindly as possible. It is no small blessing of Swami's that both of us can lead an almost normal life despite the inconveniences.

Since becoming a Sai physician, my opinion concerning the effectiveness of prayer has changed substantially. I had heard before that God is omnipresent, omniscient and omnipotent, but I saw this as a concept, not as hard fact. I believed in the historical existence of Jesus and in the good faith of the apostles who transmitted His word, but there was plenty of "noise" in the transmission. So many points remained obscure. I had a strong suspicion that lots of lessons were lost. I know, that for many people, Jesus' message is complete enough as a means to reach God but, for me it was hard to reconcile His teachings with daily life. Then Swami "appeared" on my horizon with His abundance of explanations and with His generosity to repeat these lessons adjusting the perspective to fit every audience.

In spite of twenty-nine years as a physician, I have rarely recommended to patients to address God directly. I am still hesitant to do this as I am new to trusting God myself. A nineteen-year-old girl, who has been my patient since she was born, came to see me. She was suffering from all sorts of minor ailments. She has been prone to anxiety whenever coping with responsibilities, a tendency that brought about several psychosomatic disturbances. Beginning her second year at the university, far away from home, she was having a hard time. I know her family to be Catholic with tight codes of conduct. She balked at the easygoing ways offered by our current pop culture, perhaps being too hard on herself. This resulted in a sour vision of the world, putting an extra load on her shoulders.

Before coming to Swami, I could never trust myself, but when she described her situation to me, the impulse to share with her the joy and peace I was feeling with Baba sprang into my mind. I asked her if she believed in God and, as she nodded yes, I said that He was the solution to her problems. She reacted heartily saying she knew all the theories, and they did not help. I said it was not a matter of theory but of confidence; all she had to do was trust God, then she would need no further knowledge or practice whatsoever.

I believe God made us both ripe for this exchange, because my words seemed to touch her deeply. She was instantly relieved and excited, with a broad happy smile. I met her mother a month later and then again after another six months. She proudly told me that her daughter was happy and free from any health problems.

I recall how I used to meet people at the university who were overflowing with happiness. As I replay these memories under this new light I can, at last, understand how they could have felt that way.

I want to express my gratitude to my Lord Sathya Sai Baba for healing me so that I can be a more compassionate physician and of greater service to Him. I am just beginning to experience the joy of knowing God and trusting Him. I know all of us will, one day, not only have joy but eternal life, the absolute knowledge, and perfect bliss, when we are with Him forever, and ever, and ever...

Miracles and Medicine
Venkat Kanubaddi M.D., F.A.C.A.

I was born in a small village in India in the rural state of Andhra Pradesh. We were a middle class family of farmers. Since childhood, I have always become lost in the sunset and starry night skies wondering about the mystery of creation. Though I would play with the children of the village whenever I found the opportunity, I always enjoyed solitude and contemplation.

The spirituality in our family was limited to the celebration of festivals and the worshipping of various pictures of God or idols on festival days. When I watched the villagers celebrate festivals with idol worship and sacrificing of small animals, it seemed very primitive and turned me completely away from Hinduism, which I mistook to be a religion of idol worship.

During my early years, I did not have any meaningful guidance in either worldly or spiritual matters. There was no one who could answer any of my questions. So in my own way, I took up the quest of finding out who and what God is. At the age of seven or eight, one of the converted Christians in our village told us about Jesus. I was attracted because there was no idol worship and because of Jesus' promise that He was the way and, if we come to Him, He will give us relief by bearing the burden of worldly life. So, I adopted Christianity as my path to search for God. My elder-father and elder-mother (my mother's older sister and her husband), who had adopted me, also took up Christianity. The Christian lady promised that with prayers to Jesus, my father's asthma would be healed. Though I liked Jesus' message of love, I had a problem with the concept that Jesus was the only way to reach God. Even then, in my heart, I was praying to the "Father" to whom Jesus was referring. Somehow, I had the inner knowing that there were enlightened people in other religious paths as well.

My father was a good man and, even before taking up Christianity, he used to invite different religious people to give expositions on the epics like the *Mahabharatha*. He even had a small Telugu *Bhagavad Gita* in the house. I read it page by page. Although I did not understand a lot of it, one thing was awe-inspiring. It was Lord Krishna's statement that He is the Way, the source, substance, and sustenance of this universe and, by surrendering to Him, you will gain liberation.

The question arose in my mind, "How is it that Krishna was saying the same thing as Jesus?" What is the truth? In my heart, I was happy to know that Lord Krishna was offering such a promise and that Hinduism was not just idol worship. It became very clear to me that I had to continue my search for God and truth. I felt this would be the only way to reconcile the statements of these two God men.

During one Christian convention, my father was suffering greatly from his asthma. I was praying very intensely through Jesus to "God, the Father," for relief from the severe attack. Instead of getting better, he actually passed away during the early hours of the morning. That shook my faith in Jesus and God and also brought to my awareness the temporary nature of life and relationships. My interest in Christianity began to fade. For that reason, I was never baptized.

During this time, I finished my elementary and high school education with high honors. After high school, I got admitted directly into the Medical College at Kurnool, Andhra Pradesh. The study of Embryology and the development of the fetus from two cells into one, and then multiplying to become the complex individual, were extremely fascinating to me. I could see the work of the divine hand in this. At first, I thought that science could provide the answers for my questions about God. But I soon saw the limitations of science, as its scope of inquiry was limited to the five senses. During this time, I read the revelations of a sixteenth century spiritual master who wrote about the embryological development of the fetus in the womb. How could this sage know what science has struggled so hard to find out? This baffled me. The mystical side of spirituality and its potential to reveal the truth about God, nature, and humans began to appeal to me.

After finishing my medical degree (MBBS) and surgical residency (MS) in India, I moved to the USA with my wife and two sons. Later, I completed my residency in Anesthesia (M.D.), and went into private practice. The search for God and truth always continued in spite of all the progress and accomplishments on the worldly level.

In the pursuit of truth, I studied the teachings of many masters, such as Ramakrishna Paramahamsa and Ramana Maharshi, and also met many living masters. It was at this time that I was introduced to the teachings of Vedanta, the true essence of Hinduism. The definition of God, according to Vedanta, is Prajnanam Brahma, or Consciousness is God. This really appealed to me. It was no longer Jesus, Siva, or Krishna. Through Vedanta, my inner conviction that the Cosmic Consciousness is God became very clear. The expositions of Adi Shankara about the non-dual nature to understand God, and the explanation of how the One has taken many names and forms to become the universe was fantastic. My quest for God, nature and humanity, and the relationship between them, took a quantum leap.

Although it is declared in the *Gita* that cosmic consciousness (Brahman) can take human form during different periods of time to protect dharma (righteousness), a doubt still lingered in my mind. How can the infinite power possibly be contained in some finite form and still be infinite? It was in 1987 that I came across the book *Sadhana, The Inward Path* by Sathya Sai Baba. His exposition of the concepts of Vedanta was so clear and simple that it astounded me. For this reason, I proceeded to order all the books, tapes, and everything else I could find about Him. His very simple background with meager worldly education, His mystical powers, and His knowledge of all the scriptures not only amazed me but also inspired me to explore further into this phenomenon called Sathya Sai Baba.

Up to that point, the concept in Vedanta that a person who has the knowledge of Brahman can know everything seemed metaphorical. Suddenly, the life and teachings of Sathya Sai Baba seemed to make this a real possibility. If this is so, it means that God, with all His attributes such as the power of creation, sustenance and destruction, could apparently be embodied in human form. It was very exciting to know this. I was ready to meet this God man.

During the last week of December 1990, our little angel dog, Sunshine, fell into a culvert. His hind legs became paralyzed, and he lost control of his bladder and bowel. After thorough investigation, the veterinary spine specialist could not find any surgical cause, such as fracture of the vertebrae or acute disc prolapse, that could be treated with surgery, nor could he find any medical cause such as spinal artery thrombosis. So, after three or four days of keeping him in the hospital, he gave up and suggested that we either take him home or put him to sleep. We totally ruled out the idea of putting him to sleep. My wife, our boys and myself decided to take care of him no matter what, even if it meant that I would have to work extra hard to pay for his medical expenses, as there is no such thing as canine insurance. We shed many tears for our Sunshine whom we loved so much, and he loved us all even more. All of a sudden, it occurred to me that, if Sai Baba is that cosmic power, God in human form, He could hear our prayers and help. We carried our dear Sunshine to our prayer room upstairs, placed Sai Baba's picture on the altar, and we all prayed for Sunshine's recovery. We requested that Sai Baba intervene with His grace if He was God in human form. Over the next few days, Sunshine regained his bladder and bowel functions and eventually recovered completely.

With this proof and validation, we decided to go to Puttaparthi and have Sai Baba's darshan. A few days after we arrived, in February 1991, Swami came over to me, created vibhuti and pressed it firmly with His thumb against the area of my third eye. Then, He touched my head in blessing. At that moment, I was transported to some other dimension of bliss and exhilaration. I don't know what actually happened for, by the time I came back to physical awareness, He had gone. That experience was beyond my intellectual comprehension. Before that moment, I had always believed that everything could be explained through intellectual reasoning. This showed me that there are dimensions beyond the realm of intellect that can only be experienced. On that same day, He gave padnamaskar to my wife. Thus we came into the Sai fold.

One time when He came close to me in darshan, I asked Him, "Swami, I am an anesthesiologist. When there is a need, can I have the opportunity to work in the Super Specialty Hospital?" *Yes, yes,* He replied. But I had no idea how that would come to pass, as I knew no one in the ashram or among His devotees. I wondered how I would know if I were asked to work there. But I had total faith that, somehow, He would take care of it. Subsequently, I was advised to write a letter, including my credentials, to Swami and the medical director of the Super Specialty Hospital. I was overjoyed when I was given permission to come and serve in February 1994.

After coming to Swami, miracles began to happen. I remember one day my wife asking me, "We've been on the spiritual path all along. How is it that these miracles are happening now and not before coming to Sai Baba?" I told her, "Divine grace is like sunshine. Before, we directed our prayers to the formless God. Though His blessings were there, they were not visible. God in human form is like a magnifying glass that can channel the sun's rays and bring them to a point of focus, whereby, with the heat and light, you can create fire on a piece of paper. Similarly, the avatar can channel His grace in a concentrated way to make the answers to prayers manifest more visibly. That may be the reason for visible miracles now." She smiled in agreement.

In my profession of Anesthesiology, I do cardiac, neurosurgical, and pediatric anesthesia, as well as other sub specialties. I am a senior partner in a private group practice with currently more than twenty doctors. Therefore, I get to perform all types of challenging anesthetic procedures for a variety of surgical cases.

After coming into the Sai fold, I was doing anesthesia for CAB (coronary artery bypass) on a very sick patient. His heart was functioning at about 20% ejection fraction (heart pumping capacity). The surgeon and I knew that it was going to be a difficult case. We had taken every precaution and were prepared to deal with anything that could happen. After completing the coronary artery grafts, the surgeon tried to wean the patient from the heart-lung machine (the pump). It was unsuccessful. So, he put an intra aortic balloon pump to help the failing heart's pumping action, and I added several pharmacological drips to support the function of the heart. Still, the heart was not able to sustain the blood pressure. He put the patient back on the pump while we were thinking aloud about the other possibilities that could help with this situation. If our efforts didn't succeed, there was a possibility that the patient would die on the operating table.

The surgeon told me that he was going to check all the grafts to see if he could find a problem. He had already done this once before, and all the grafts had looked fine. I couldn't add any more medicine, as I was already on the maximum dosage with all the drips. So while the surgeon was checking the grafts, I put my right hand on the patient's forehead, closed my eyes and prayed to Sai Baba. "Dear Sai, only Your grace can turn things around here. All our human efforts are failing. If this patient and his family deserve Your grace, please intervene and help." At that point, the surgeon said that the grafts were all okay and, again, requested that we attempt to wean the patient from the pump. Amazingly, this time, as we continued the weaning, the blood pressure held steady instead of dropping. Finally, we were successful in weaning, and the blood pressure stayed around 110/70. The surgeon looked at the monitors and then looked at me in disbelief thinking that I had adjusted the drips to make things better. He said, "Venkat, what miracle have you done? Everything looks great." I replied, "I have done nothing different except pray. God has answered our prayers, that is all." The mood in the operating room was once again joyful. I silently thanked Swami, as I knew that it was His grace that had made the difference for the patient.

It is in the direst and most hopeless situations that Swami's grace and power to intervene become most apparent. In August 1998, a young man in his mid forties suffered from a major heart attack. His wife and little daughter, not the patient, occasionally came to our Sai Center.   One night, in the early hours of the morning, he had severe chest discomfort. His brother, who is a cardiologist, took him to the emergency room and got him admitted to the hospital. Upon heart catheterization, they found severely obstructed arteries to the heart, and so they scheduled an emergency coronary artery bypass (CAB).

The surgery took much longer than expected, and he was on the heart-lung machine for 3-4 hours. This is a very long time compared to the normal CAB. While weaning him from the heart-lung machine, the anesthesiologist and the surgeon had to use several drips and the aortic balloon pump to support the heart. Subsequently, he was put on a respirator in the ICU. This is done routinely for such cases. However, unlike routine CAB cases, on the following day the patient was unable to be weaned from the respirator. He was a heavy smoker, and the doctors thought that this might be the reason for the delay.

Over the next several days, his lungs got even worse, and he had to be left on the ventilator and kept sedated. Meanwhile his kidneys began to fail, and he had to be placed on kidney dialysis. When his liver functions were checked, they looked bad. Subsequently he developed ischemia of the bowel and had to be taken for emergency surgery to remove the dead bowel. As the lung condition was not improving, he had to be given a tracheotomy for long-term ventilation. Whenever I went to see this patient at the hospital, he was incoherent and thrashing around. Therefore, he had to be restrained and continually sedated. As his neurological condition was also deteriorating, they did a CT scan of the brain that showed infarction of the brain. It meant some of the brain function could be lost forever even if he survived.

The look of desperation on the face of his wife was heart wrenching. Many people making different comments about the outcome of this case added to her anguish. At our Sai Center, we all offered our prayers to Swami on behalf of this patient and his family. His little daughter, who had absolute faith in Swami, would say, "Sai Baba is God. He alone can help daddy."

At that time, my wife and I had to make an emergency trip to India, and so we went to Prashanthi Nilayam to have Swami's darshan. I wrote a letter to Swami about this patient and also about the predicament of the wife and the little daughter. As I was holding the letter in my hand, Swami came close, gave me padnamaskar, looked at the letter intently and took it. The next day, when we called Fort Wayne to talk to our friends and inquire about this patient, they mentioned that, the night before, the patient deteriorated so badly that everyone gave up hope. However, today things were looking a little better. I mentioned to them about Swami acknowledging our prayer and taking the letter and asked them to inform the family about this. They were not to lose hope.

We returned to Fort Wayne four or five days later. Upon our arrival, I went to the hospital to see the patient. His wife narrated all the critical developments including the night when they totally lost hope. When we tallied the dates, it was about the same time that Swami accepted the letter. The following morning, he had looked a bit more stable. I reassured her that, since Swami accepted the letter of prayer, He would intervene. I encouraged her to continue to pray and keep the faith. I gave her Swami's holy ash to apply to her husband's forehead. A smile of hope flashed on her lips. In the face of the gloomy prognosis forecast by the doctors and everyone else, this was probably the only word of hope and reassurance she had been given.

Amazingly, things started to get better. Over the next week, his lungs started to improve. He could be weaned off the respirator. His kidney functions improved, and dialysis could be discontinued over the next several days. He began to respond appropriately to his wife, daughter and family. When I went to visit him, he recognized me and thanked all of us for our prayers. Over the next two to three weeks, he started eating well and gained enough strength to be discharged home.

It is now a year later, and you could never tell that he was the same person who was on his deathbed with all the bodily systems failing, including his brain. This is truly a medical miracle. It astonished every doctor involved in the management of this case. This is the divine power of Sai intervening with His grace.

I always had great interest in understanding human diseases and the process of healing. To facilitate this understanding, I took medical training in Maharishi Ayurveda. I have also had the opportunity to serve as the Medical Director for a holistic healing center called the Wellness Oasis in Fort Wayne, Indiana. These experiences, along with various interviews with Sathya Sai Baba, gave me some insight into the reasons for illnesses and the process of healing.

Diseases come from three different levels: body, conscious mind and unconscious mind. Though diseases can originate at any of these three levels, quite frequently the manifestation can be at the body level. The causes for diseases at the body level are due to polluted foods, water, air, bacteria, viruses and wrong living habits, such as smoking, drinking alcohol and living out of tune with the rhythms of nature. The causes of the diseases of the conscious mind are generally due to stressful living at work and home, lack of love and understanding in relationships, no understanding of the purpose of life, and being overpowered by the negative emotions of greed, jealousy, pride, anger, lust and attachment.

The diseases that originate at the deep unconscious level of the mind are the genetic disorders, autoimmune disorders, cancer and so forth, which in turn are due to negative karma carried over from previous lives or acquired during the earlier part of this lifetime. These illnesses can manifest at the conscious mind or body level, though they actually originate at the deepest level.

The treatment for bodily illnesses is best accomplished with the help of modern Allopathic Medicine with all its advanced diagnostic and therapeutic methods. The treatment for illnesses of the conscious mind can be accomplished through stress free living and re-establishing love as the theme for all relationships. Healing for the illnesses at the unconscious mind level, due to negative karma, can be accomplished by invoking divine grace through prayer, faith, selfless service and right moral living (practicing truth, right conduct, peace, love and nonviolence). That is why, sometimes, after trying and exhausting all other methods, devotees with terminal illnesses will come to Swami and be healed by His mere touch or look. That is the power of God working from the deepest and innermost level.

In 1997, a long time devotee of Sai Baba was diagnosed with severe CAD (Coronary Artery Disease). He had plenty of financial resources and so wanted to come to the USA to have his operation. However, his wife, being a very ardent devotee, wanted Baba's blessings before doing anything. To answer her prayers, Baba spoke to them and told them to have CAB (Coronary Artery Bypass) done in Parthi at the Super Specialty Hospital and not in the USA. By Swami's will, I was chosen to give the anesthetic, and a cardiac surgeon from the USA was chosen to perform the surgery.

On the day of the surgery, Swami came to the operating room, blessed the patient while he was laying on the table and, then, with His hand on my head, blessed me and touched the chain around my neck that he had previously created. Then He went out and sat on a chair watching everything through the glass door. Induction of anesthetic went very smoothly, and everything was very stable. I went out to report this and take padnamaskar. While I was taking padnamaskar, Swami blessed me on my head and said, *During the procedure, watch the blood pressure and blood sugar carefully.*

Lo and behold, once we went on to the pump, his blood pressure (BP) started to go all over the place. It slid down to zero, and my attempt to bring it up with medications didn't have much impact. Very much concerned, I started to invoke Baba's grace through prayer and, in my mind, I began reciting the Sai Gayatri. Then the blood pressure started to come up, but it went up in the other direction to more than 250/120. Again, my attempts to reduce it with medications failed, and I again resorted to prayer and the Sai Gayatri. The blood pressure responded and came down, but then it would go in the other direction. This seesaw business was going on for quite some time. Meanwhile, the surgeon, oblivious to all this, was doing bypass grafts. Gradually, the blood pressure swings became less and less as the surgeon got close to completing the grafts. At the same time, the blood sugar also went up very high, and I had to use insulin on the heart lung machine to bring it down to acceptable levels. Subsequently, the surgery was completed, the patient stabilized, and we were able to wean him from the heart-lung machine without much difficulty.

However, I still had my own concerns about the outcome. I felt there was a good chance of this patient developing hemiplegia (paralysis of one side of the body) due to his extremely high BP (blood pressure), or substantial memory loss due to his dangerously low BP with no blood flow to the brain for a brief period of time. The proof of the outcome would be when he woke up in the ICU (Intensive Care Unit). Hence, I watched him very closely.

He woke up from the anesthetic in less than two hours and was able to be extubated (removing the breathing tube through which the respirator delivers O2). Right after extubation, he seemed very alert and was offering to me "Namaste," with folded palms, as an act of thankfulness. I pointed him towards Swami's photo and asked him to offer thanks to Him. I was very happy to see the movement of all his limbs and also the clarity of mind. I again offered my prayer of gratitude to Swami for His intervention. It took a few days to stabilize his blood sugar, but with close monitoring of blood sugar and adjustment of insulin dosage, his recovery was complete without complications.

During my twenty years of practicing Anesthesiology, I had never witnessed such BP swings in heart surgery. I knew that it was the grace of Swami that saved this devotee from major complications, because none of my medications worked in time. This is an example of health problems, due to bad karma, that could be reversed by divine grace.

Another experience of divine grace at the Super Specialty Hospital was in 1994. The visiting cardiologist, from our USA group, requested that I be available for resuscitation in case the angioplasty (balloon dilatation of coronary arteries) got into trouble. The patient scheduled for this procedure had a heart that functioned very poorly and could not withstand surgery. However, if he should get into trouble during angioplasty due to a tear in the artery or the dislodging of plaque, it could lead to a major heart attack or, possibly, death. The only way to save him would be to do emergency heart surgery, which itself could cause death. For this reason, he asked me to be there to resuscitate in case of problems and to avoid emergency surgery.

The coronary artery that he had to dilate was very tortuous. He had to first pass a guide wire and then send a small balloon catheter over it and dilate the narrowed artery. The artery was so twisted and narrow that he could not negotiate the wire. He didn't want to force it for fear of rupturing or dissecting the vessel or dislodging the plaque. So, he stopped the procedure for a while. At this point, we all decided to pray for Baba's help. We all chanted "Sai Ram" three times. Then, the cardiologist attempted to pass the guide wire again. This time, it passed through very smoothly. He was able to advance the balloon catheter over it and dilate the narrow portion in a few minutes. Everybody was extremely happy as everything went without a hitch.

The next morning, when we were at darshan, Swami came nearby, looked at us and said, *Yesterday evening, you had problems with the catheter and had to call on Swami. Swami had to come to the rescue.* We all felt extremely happy to hear those words. They confirmed to us that when we selflessly pray, God does hear our prayers and does shower grace to avoid calamities and complications. This is a clear example of Swami's omnipresence.

After coming into the fold of the avatar, the embodiment of divine love, my life and my medical practice changed. Though I was a vegetarian until I entered medical college, I succumbed to peer-pressure and began to eat meat during my college days. After Swami, I was able to revert back to being a vegetarian without much difficulty. I have also become more careful in watching my thoughts, speech and actions, as I know that Swami is always witnessing everything. I do this by being true to my inner self, which is Swami. Even while I am working or undertaking other duties to the very best of my ability, I remember the name of Sai in the back of my mind at all times, either by repeating the Sai name or remembering a Sai bhajan. This brings me a lot of peace, because I am less caught up in the dramas of the ego.

Since coming to Swami, I have certainly become more compassionate and understanding of my patient's anxieties and fears; and therefore, can offer them solace and reassurance. One of my surgical colleagues introduces me to his patients saying, "This is the kindest doctor in Fort Wayne and an excellent anesthesiologist." I feel this compliment really belongs to Swami and not to me. It is Swami who brought out these qualities.

Before my patients undergo surgery, I suggest that they pray. While speaking to them, I invoke Swami's grace, through a mental prayer, and bless my patients, asking for a quick restoration of good health. In tune with the principle of holistic healing, I bring their minds to a state of calmness and cheerfulness before letting them ease into the anesthetic. I play gentle music while giving subliminal messages that the outcome will be wonderful. I make sure that nobody in the operating room, thinking that the patient is asleep, talks negatively about the outcome. After surgery, almost all the patients report to me that they had a very good anesthetic experience. That gives me a lot of job satisfaction, and I always offer a prayer of gratitude to Swami for His guidance and help. I believe it is very important to invoke divine guidance and blessings before a procedure. By shifting the responsibility from our own shoulders to God, we can really enjoy the work.

Swami has also brought to the forefront the attitude of selfless service. I now offer service in a free heath clinic and, along with members of our Sai Center in the Fort Wayne area, serve the elderly, disabled and hungry. With Swami's grace, it has been possible to establish a high school building for the children in our native village in India. They have implemented the EHV (Education in Human Values) Program into the school system. It has also been possible to establish an industry in rural Telangana, a poverty-stricken area of Andhra Pradesh, to provide jobs for the deserving poor. Swami made it possible for our family to sponsor the education of some orphaned children in India. He has also given me an opportunity to volunteer my services in the Super Specialty Hospital in Parthi. Swami is never tired of reminding us that service to God is really through service to our fellow human beings and all the creatures in the universe.

The miracles in medicine can inspire us to search for answers and to understand the healing process within the complex human being. The actual healing happens when the divine energy of the atma flows unimpeded through the various sheaths and brings wholeness to each sheath: the physical, the physiological, the emotional, the intellectual, and the bliss sheath. Physicians are only the facilitators. The patient and the physician can work together to remove the obstacles to the free flow of the divine energy. This is done through a combination of modern allopathic medicine and holistic medicines such as Ayurveda and Homeopathy. Divine grace, invoked through prayer and combined with the above medical systems, can make perfect health possible.

This understanding brings a great deal of excitement and inspiration into my medical practice and enables me to really rejoice in my work. My work feels as if it is the worship of God, and I feel the blessings that come from such work. As I contemplate all these transforming events of my life, these words of Swami keep ringing in my ears:

> *Duty without Love is Deplorable.*
> *Duty with Love is Desirable.*
> *Love without Duty is Divine.*

God is Love
Franco Pluchino, M.D.

I heard Sai Baba's name mentioned for the first time about twenty years ago. I was in a restaurant in northern Italy with a group of friends. We were keen to try the famous polenta with cheese, which is a specialty of the area, and we had heard that an excellent cook ran this restaurant. We were all in a very good mood, talking and laughing, enjoying good food and wine. Then, suddenly, in the middle of the meal, someone said something that prompted a colleague of mine to talk about his trip to India and his meeting with a great spiritual master in whom he had perceived the divine essence. He told us he had become a devotee of this holy man called Sai Baba. He spoke about what a fascinating being He was, how He walked every morning among thousands of devotees from all over the world who were seated silently on the ground. He told us how they gazed, mesmerized, at this being who materialized sacred ash from His hand while He walked among several thousand people collecting letters. Some people reached out begging Him to fulfill their wishes. He went on to tell us about Sai Baba's teachings on the meaning of our existence and of the great love that we should all develop towards our fellow beings.

What struck me most about this was my colleague's utter devotion for Sai Baba. When he finished his story, he extracted from his wallet a tiny envelope containing the sacred ash, called vibhuti, which he showed us with a glazed look in his eye. While he was talking, I had kept resolutely quiet; but in the end, I exploded saying that I was convinced he was not only quite crazy but also suffering from some form of senility.

Although raised in a deeply religious Catholic family, over the years I had become a hard-core atheist and had long abandoned any religious convictions. My scientific career had also reinforced my atheism. It was impossible to accept something which did not offer a rational explanation. It was, therefore, totally irrational to contemplate the idea of God becoming a man in order to save humanity. I, for one, needed no intermediary for my salvation. My strong reaction was perfectly normal to me. Indian gurus were very much in fashion at the time, and it was madness to describe any of them as divine incarnations. The debate became quite heated, almost out of control, so we decided it was better to move to other topics and not upset our digestion.

However, in the following days, I could not get the thought out of my mind that my colleague, who was such an intelligent person, a professional held in high esteem by all, could lose his critical faculties and be so easily taken in by a so-called Indian holy man. I searched frantically for a rational explanation to this behavior but could find none.

Several years passed before I heard again about Sai Baba. My wife, who had been present at the famous polenta meal and had taken part in the discussion, but in a much more subdued way, told me that she had been watching an English program on TV about Sai Baba. She added that she had been rather surprised by the presentation of this strange being who lived in an ashram in South India, because the comments were very fair and devoid of sarcasm. They were showing Sai Baba walking amidst thousands of people who had come from all over the world to see Him.

After some years went by, we were invited to India for a seminar. At the end of it, we decided to go on an extended tour of Northern and Central India. The wealth and artistic monuments deeply impressed us. We were struck by the massive crowds of people who, though living in extreme poverty and performing heavy and tiring daily work, especially in large urban areas, seemed to be quite serene. We were also fascinated by the Indian landscape's intense colors and by the beautiful colored saris the women wore with such elegance, moving about like fashion models. But what my wife and I both felt, in spite of our lack of spirituality, was the aura of spirituality that pervaded the Indian temples and the Indian people whom we met.

We fully enjoyed this trip, which took us daily to beautiful places though, from time to time, we would inexplicably feel drawn to inquire of some Indian: "Do you know Sai Baba?" Or, "Do you know where Sai Baba lives?" We did not get any satisfactory answer, because either they had not heard of Him, or they did not want to tell us about Him. We went back home with beautiful memories of India, hoping to return again. But for some years this wish did not materialize.

Back home, I resumed my work and my daily routine. One day, a woman with her two daughters came to see me. She had already been to my office, and I had performed an examination which had revealed a benign but large tumor in the brain. Reluctantly, I advised her on the necessity of a surgical intervention. There was no other solution. However, it was quite obvious, even to someone without any medical knowledge, that such an intervention was not without risks. I was, therefore, expecting, as generally happens, an anxious reaction from her. I was quite surprised to hear this lady tell me with a bright smile: "Professor, if you must operate, please go ahead and do it as soon as possible."

A few days later, she was operated on and, when it was over, I went to speak to her husband and daughters who, with great anxiety, were waiting for me. I told them I was quite satisfied and expressed confidence that there would be no sequel. Everything happened as expected. The next day, the patient was fully conscious and able to communicate with us.

After the morning visit, the assistant who had helped me during the operation said: "Do you know that this lady is a Sai Baba devotee?" He had been with us in India and had participated in our search for Sai Baba. I was quite happy to hear this news, and it awakened in me the desire to know more about this strange man whose name had cropped up a few times in the past. I had the opportunity to question my patient, Paola, many times during her stay in the hospital. She was always very happy to talk about Him and did so with the greatest devotion. I was, however, shocked when she confided one day to me: "I must tell you something quite important. The night before the operation, I saw Sai Baba next to me. He was wearing His usual orange robe and told me, 'Don't worry, everything will be fine. I will be guiding your surgeon's hands.'" When I came out of her room, I said to my assistant: "Oh dear! I'm afraid I have done something quite wrong to Paola's brain!"

However, our discussions continued, and I learned that, before their marriage, her husband had spent six years living in the ashram. My curiosity was aroused. I asked her if I could meet her husband and hear more about his experience. A few months later, when Paola came back to the clinic for a checkup, she was accompanied by her husband. Francesco is someone who immediately inspires confidence. His eyes gleam with intelligence; what he says is fascinating; and he is always happy to hear your comments. He spoke of his long stay at the ashram, of the joy of living close to such a great spiritual master who transforms and drives us on spiritually, helping us know the purpose of our existence. He told me how Sai Baba offers a teaching, based on love, to help us realize our inner divinity. This love must extend to all, enemies or friends, irrespective of their religions as religions are many, but God is only one.

He also spoke of his task during those years. He used to help Italians who, arriving daily in droves to this insignificant Indian hamlet and unable to speak any English, came with one aim only: to see Sai Baba, listen to him, and be close to Him. Though Francesco spoke with great passion, I was not particularly touched. I was, nevertheless, listening with great attention and interest. I was also somewhat curious to learn more about this odd man who, for many years, kept coming up in my life in one way or another. I was even tempted to go back to India. So, finally, I asked Francesco if I could join him for his next trip. He cordially replied: "When you decide to go, just let me know. I will be very happy if you will join us. My wife and I usually go there at least once a year."

The following months confirmed the divergence between thoughts and actions. The good intention was there, but I did not do anything about it, though Francesco called me twice when they were leaving for Puttaparthi. Unfortunately, I had a busy schedule each time and was not free. When he called me the third time, however, I decided to go and to drop all my commitments. So, I told him that both my wife and I would join them and to let me know the date.

We were quite excited by the prospect of going to Puttaparthi and took great care in the preparation, sticking meticulously to Paola's list of suggestions. When the plane took off, we were both convinced that this was going to be a very unusual experience, not to be missed for the world. When we landed in Bangalore, we had to take a taxi to our destination, approximately three hours away, across the Indian countryside. The trip itself was a sheer delight. The landscape was beautiful with enormous palm trees and banana plantations, and we noticed a strong light that seemed to permeate everything around us. We traveled through quaint small villages. The walls of the huts consisted of a mixture of mud, wood and metal. Lining both sides of the road were rows of tiny shops selling fruit, drinks and clothing. There were also repair shops right in the middle of the road. Just before arriving at our destination, Puttaparthi, we saw some of Sai Baba's wonderful constructions: the new hospital with 300 beds, a superb building where heart operations are being carried out completely free of charge. Adjacent is the Puttaparthi Airport where many devotees arrive daily. Also, we saw a university, schools, and a planetarium.

At the entrance of the town was a big arch welcoming all. Then, we reached the ashram, a very large area, where Sai Baba's mandir (temple) stands majestically in the center. This is where the devotees gather to attend Sai Baba's daily darshan. There are also many colorful buildings housing numberless devotees.

I was immediately struck by the quiet and serene atmosphere, especially noticeable when compared to the chaos we had just left behind. There were many westerners. Men were wearing white pajamas. Some women wore saris and others long dresses or outfits that seemed like pajamas. The next morning, we were up at four o'clock as agreed, and I joined the other men while my wife joined the women, as is the rule in the ashram. There were thousands of people, all queuing up in total silence outside the temple, waiting to be allowed inside. Then we entered in orderly rows guided to our places by attendants. I was spellbound. Here were, literally, thousands of people ready to sit on the ground with their legs crossed, very close to each other, for long hours and in total silence. Many were Indian, but there were also many from other countries. I was looking around thinking, "These people are either mad or fanatics." I kept looking with no other thought but what was taking place in front of my eyes. A few hours went by when I suddenly heard some music, and I saw people straightening up their backs and looking in a certain direction. Then Sai Baba appeared. I saw in the distance a small man with a crown of black, frizzy hair, wearing an orange robe. He was walking very slowly in the middle of this crowd of seated people while gathering letters handed to Him by devotees whose faces expressed pure joy. My eyes followed him for a while, and then I thought, "All this is absurd! But who is this guy? Where does he come from? What am I doing here? I must be as mad as the rest. I wonder what my nurses would say if they saw me here."

I remembered that, one day, the nurses confessed to me that they had stuck the image of a saint under my operating room chair, because I was often in the habit of swearing badly during surgery. The nurses used to pray softly when I swore saying, "Please Lord, forgive him, as he does not know what he is saying!" What I was doing now was, therefore, absurd, thinking about my nurses and the saint under the seat. An atheist in a monastery! When Sai Baba came closer, I realized He was much smaller and more fragile than I had first thought. After about half an hour or less, He disappeared into his rooms followed by some of the devotees He had selected for an interview.

My reaction to this first meeting was one of skepticism. I was certainly not enthusiastic. Francesco sensed this and told me again what he had said many times before: "Don't pay attention to your feelings now. Let a few days pass." I told him I trusted him and would follow his advice. After the darshan, we got up to go back to our room. As usual, Francesco was walking with a brisk step, and I was following him. We were both immersed in our own thoughts, walking in silence. I could only think of this morning's events which I had found most peculiar, to say the least. As for Francesco, he was probably overcome by the strong emotion of the vision of Baba that surged in him each time he saw Him.

All of a sudden, a young man in his thirties, heavily built and prematurely bald stopped me exclaiming: "Professor! You here too?" He looked both surprised and happy. "I am an assistant doctor in the neuro-surgery department at Bologna's hospital. I have seen you many times at our seminars." I replied that I was very happy to meet him. Somehow I felt compelled to justify: "I have come here with a friend, but it's my first visit to Puttaparthi, and I am not a devotee of Sai Baba." But my young friend replied with great conviction: "I understand; but if you are here, it is because Sai Baba has called you. You will see. From now on, your life will change. It happened to me several years ago."

I did not want to upset him by telling him I did not share his conviction, so I changed the subject and said how favorably impressed I was by the atmosphere in the ashram. We finally parted company hoping to meet up again. I had just gone a few steps when he rushed back to me and said, "Professor, can I tell my friends at the hospital that I met you here?" I was slightly taken aback by his request, but replied smiling: "Of course! Do so. I have nothing to hide." Satisfied by my answer, he went away.

On the second day, my feelings were unchanged, and my disappointment grew even bigger. But on the third day, something happened that changed my life. This time, we were quite lucky. We were sitting right in front, in the first line. I would be able to see Him more closely. As soon as I heard the music signaling his appearance, I kept looking at Him, watching every movement as He was coming closer and closer. Then He was in front of me, looking at me. His piercing glance penetrated into me. It was incredibly powerful, but also incredibly gentle. How long did it last? I do not know. It seemed an eternity. His eyes were locked in mine. It was just the two of us! A feeling of intense happiness and emotion surged in me. I was in some kind of a trance, with my eyes fixed on Him, while he was moving away. I realized instantly that my life had changed. Francesco's voice brought me back to earth. "Wow! Amazing! What a look He gave you!"

When I told my wife what had happened, I could see that she, too, had noticed a change in me. Her inclination, as a non-believer, had also undergone some change, albeit not as strong as mine.

In the following days, I had long conversations with Francesco about the meaning of life. "Life, life! It's only illusion," Francesco was saying. "We are here to realize ourselves, the divinity within, and the only possible way is through love." I spent many hours in the mandir area thinking about my life, my profession, for which I had a great passion, my social activities, my fights against injustice and suffering, and my love for my family. I was mostly concerned with finding an answer to the meaning of our existence. What before had been my life's objective, helping man to progress and the defense of ethical values, now no longer seemed to satisfy me. Previously, death meant the physical decay of the body, where the soul played no part. Now I wasn't so sure about that. What I had always believed now seemed very limited and did not provide an answer to the many questions about life. I had often wondered, for instance, why I had to watch the suffering and, sometimes, death of young children or young people with brain tumors and be totally powerless. If God did exist, was He so merciless that He allowed such suffering to take place?

I found the answers in Sai Baba's teachings. We reap the consequences of deeds in previous incarnations; and therefore, each life follows its own course. What is important, then, is to tread the path in this life which will lead you to identify yourself with the divinity inside. Death is not a tragic event but, rather, the beginning of something new that could lead to Self-realization.

I was immersed in these new thoughts which had never crossed my mind before. I was trying to adapt myself to these new ideas. In the mornings, when I watched Baba amongst the crowds, I knew He was the one who could help me. I was reading over and over again what Baba has said: *I have called you here in order to see you, and that you should see Me. In this look and*

*vision I have granted you lies your transformation which will be
accelerated, intensified, and increased. I am revealing Myself to
you so you should know Me. Even if you think I take no notice of
you, I am the one who has called you here.*

After these ten days in Puttaparthi which had such an impact
on my life, as well as my wife's, we returned to Italy. A change in
our lives is normally understood as a positive change, for instance
in the way we live, a change in our job, an improvement in our
working conditions, a higher salary, or a change in our well
being, either financial or physical. By 'change' we generally
mean an external modification, not an inner one, which could
lead us to view life and death differently from the vision we
entertained previously. My change, due to meeting a Supreme
Being, resulted in my becoming aware of my divine essence. This
transformation did not express itself in my work as a surgeon, as I
had always carried out this task as humanly as possible but,
rather, in my relationship with the people around me, whether
they were good and pleasant or bad and unpleasant. My social
work had always led me to fight against abuse of power and
injustice. I understood now that all individuals have the ability to
improve themselves through love. There was in me a strong
desire to change though I recognized that it would be a difficult
task to bridge the gap between my desire to change and the will to
do it.

When I went back to work, my colleagues and my nurses
welcomed me, eager to hear about the trip. I told them quite
frankly what had happened to me. They were so amazed that I felt
like laughing, "Franco! What are you saying? You, telling us all
these things? Do you realize how much you have changed?" They
pestered me to tell them the story again and again, and I never
had the slightest doubt that they were totally convinced that what
I was telling them was perfectly true. "We believe what you say
only because we know you," they said. Some even added, "I am
tempted to go there and see what you have seen."

In the family circle, reactions were similar. I have two
daughters whom I love and who love and esteem me. They did
not have a religious upbringing as we were lay people, but we

taught them ethical values. They were astonished by the account of my visit, by my vision of Sai Baba as a Supreme Being who is able to know our past, and by my wife's and my strong desire to practice His teachings. We wanted to lead a life fully aware that all that surrounds us is an illusion that prevents us from reaching the final objective: union with the divine. It was certainly not easy for them to accept this total transformation in our way of thinking. It was interesting to notice that people reacted in two different ways to the same story. In some, there was the curiosity to learn more and to experiment; and in others, indifference or rejection.

At work there was, however, a notable change. As I said before, I had always tried to be sympathetic and understanding with staff and patients, and this of course did not change. What did change, though, was my behavior at the operating table. Previously, I never felt the desire to ask for God's help or utter a magical formula before an operation. After my return from Puttaparthi, and on the eve of an operation, I started to appeal to Sai Baba to guide me. I felt very serene afterwards.

I recall one instance when I had to operate on a young man. The operation was particularly difficult. I was very concerned. Whereas before, I would have been swearing profusely, this time I turned to Sai Baba for help. Everything went well but, when he woke up and I checked his neurological condition, I realized that he was partly paralyzed. I became very anxious wondering what would happen to this young man and if and where I had made a mistake. All night, I prayed asking Sai Baba to save him. I was totally immersed in this new way of thinking and had completely forgotten my atheism. The first thing I did in the morning was to call the hospital and see how the patient was faring. I was told that he had regained full consciousness and the use of his limbs. During my long career, I have never witnessed such a quick and total recovery in the case of a paralysis. I had no doubt, whatsoever, that Baba had performed a miracle. When I mentioned this incident to my daughter, who is also a neuro-surgeon, she was puzzled. She admitted, though, that it was indeed an exceptional recovery.

There is another example where my faith in Baba helped me. I had programmed for the afternoon a very difficult operation. I woke up that morning with a bad migraine. I was prone to migraines, but this one was particularly strong. I tried every medicine I had to no avail. I knew that it would stay with me all day, and it would be a big problem. Early in the afternoon, I turned to Sai Baba and massaged my temples with vibhuti. A little later, I went to the clinic with the intention of postponing the operation. But when I arrived there, I had forgotten what I had intended to do and asked that the patient be sent to the operating theater. When the eight long hours were over, and the patient had regained consciousness, I suddenly remembered my awful migraine. I had completely forgotten about it. I had put the vibhuti on long after I had taken the medicine, which had had no effect. I had not realized, until later, that it was the vibhuti that was responsible for the disappearance of the migraine. I was grateful to Sai Baba for the help he had given my patient and me.

The simplicity and depth of Sai Baba's teachings are no doubt the only path that will lead us closer to Him. They have also led me to change my usual reading material, which used to be mainly historical and political books. I realized that they could not enrich me spiritually. His discourses offer a wealth of knowledge and truths. We should not look on these as a mere intellectual exercise, because this is profound spiritual material. We are lucky to have so many records of the words of the divine.

As time passed, I became nostalgic about this far away country where, every day, one can be close to Swami, where the days are spent forgetting the outside world, where one lives so peacefully, where the hours pass in such intense spiritual concentration that time itself seems to vanish. When people ask us what we do when we go to India, it is so difficult to explain.

A year later, we returned to Puttaparthi. We were, as before, a group of four with a few other devotees joining us. This trip, too, consolidated my belief in the divine essence. I was also very happy because Sai Baba always took the letters I handed to him. While sitting at darshan, I thought about Baba who, in His great love for his devotees, appears for darshan twice every single day.

When I see Him appearing daily, alone, with such simplicity, I cannot help thinking of the superficial rites of other religions. I was also struck by all His knowledge concerning events, emotions, and the reaction of people from other cultures. But I realized immediately that my thinking was incorrect. I realized that the reason He knew about everyone was because He is omnipresent and omniscient. While waiting for Baba, I was watching His students and the way they were behaving. I thought that, here, in front of my eyes, are the future leaders of India.

After seven months, without my wife this time, I returned to India for the third time. During this trip, something marvelous happened. Because thousands of devotees throng daily into the ashram, there is very little hope of getting an interview with Sai Baba. We were a large group of Italian devotees led by Ampelio, one of the nicest men I have ever met. He has been very close to Sai Baba and has talked to him many times. He was responsible for the kitchen during our time there, and we were helping him. This meant going to the kitchen at 2 a.m., peeling potatoes and other vegetables, making tons of pizzas, washing all the kitchen equipment and utensils, and serving the devotees three times a day. It was a job we all carried out with much enthusiasm and joy, as strong bonds of friendship united us. It was also a service that Sai Baba surely appreciated. We attended the darshans with great devotion but, though I was very much aware of the ardent desire of devotees to be granted an interview, I did not feel the same urge. I thought it was highly unlikely this would happen. To me, just seeing Sai Baba was like having an interview. Anyway, I felt it was better to think in this way rather than be disappointed.

It was July 11th, 1998 and only a few days remained. I was in the mandap, immersed in my thoughts after Baba had walked by. My friends suddenly brought me back to reality. "Go! Go!" they shouted, "Baba has called your group." I rushed to the door where Baba holds His interviews. When I approached to enter, He tapped me very firmly on the shoulder and told me with the sweetest smile, *You are the brain surgeon!* It is impossible to describe what I felt, as I was dazed and not really aware of what was happening. I went into the small room where there were about fifteen people seated closely together on the floor. Having recovered from the initial shock, I thought, "Baba has built a very big hospital, big schools, big universities. but for Him, this small space is enough." After a few minutes, Baba came in. He was so close, and it seemed as if we had been friends forever. He was telling us where to sit. Then with a big sigh, He went to the wall facing His armchair and turned on the fan, exclaiming, *It is very hot here!* I thought to myself, "Here is Sai Baba, alone, a simple man, a small man, and an avatar; yet here He is without a court of ministers and secretaries."

Although we were all sweating profusely, His face did not show one drop of sweat. He talked to us explaining the problems of some of the people in the room. One had a problem with his father, another a difficult marriage, another was sick and needed to be comforted in his faith. They were all completely surprised and nodding in agreement. After talking with all of us, the private interviews began. Baba took the people He selected into the adjacent room to talk to them. After a few interviews, He beckoned for my friend and me to come inside. It was just the two of us, alone, in front of Sai Baba. What happened is difficult for me to describe. A strong emotion swelled up inside, and I was no longer completely aware of what was happening. I know that Sai Baba started to advise my friend to become more involved with his work. I had to translate for my friend who kept on repeating, "It's true! It's true!" Then I spoke about the experience I had when He first glanced at me during my first visit, when I was still an atheist. Baba looked at me gently saying, *I know. I know.* I told him of my wish to work in His hospital, and He answered, *Oh, yes. Next time.* I do not know what else He said, because I was too dazed. I could only think that, here I was in front of God. I was fully convinced of this, and I can still remember this feeling perfectly. I also remember that I showed Him my grandson's picture, and He touched it lightly saying, *He is a lovely child.* At the end of the interview, He asked my friend what he wanted, and my friend replied, "Baba, Your light." Baba waved His hand and a ring with a diamond appeared, seemingly, out of nowhere. Baba slipped the ring on his finger, and it was clear my friend was overcome with emotion.

When we returned to the outer room, our friends told us that it was clear from the expression on our faces, that we had had a profound experience. We stayed a little longer with Baba and saw another materialization, one for a very sick person in our group. I saw, right in front of my eyes, a japamala drop out horizontally from His palm. This was against the law of gravity. He then caught it and put around the person's neck. At the end of the interview, He took a plastic shopping bag containing small envelopes of vibhuti and, generously and happily, distributed them. For someone who manifests gold rings and precious stones, this humble vibhuti bag underlined Sai Baba's humility.

If you asked me who I met coming out of the interview room, I could not tell you. I only remember meeting Ampelio, when I went to the kitchen for my nightly duties. We hugged each other and burst into tears. For days and days, when someone asked me to tell them about the interview, I could not speak. I was too overcome by emotion, with tears coming to my eyes. Even today, more than a year after the event, my emotion is as intense as before. I am still filled with the vivid memories of these unforgettable moments.

We came back from this trip saturated with the joy that Swami had given us so freely and decided on the spot to return in December. And so it happened. But this time, besides my wife, my younger daughter, who lives in California, also joined us. She was touched by the change she had witnessed in her parents. She, too, must have been called by Baba because something strange happened to her. The first time she attended darshan she commented on the lovely scent emanating from Baba. Both her mother and Paola, who were seated next to her, had noticed nothing. A few days later, she came with joy to tell me that Baba had taken her letters. Her happiness was so great that I felt she, too, was bound to Baba by love.

From the moment I realized that Baba had transformed my life and expanded my spiritual consciousness, I have thought about the changes this meeting has brought to my scientific outlook and my profession as a surgeon. I had always considered science as an amalgamation of unexplained natural phenomena. In the field of medical science, in particular, each new discovery is valid after repeated tests have confirmed its validity. It has, therefore, been difficult to reconcile my old thought patterns to Sai Baba's so-called "miracles." Like most lay people, I had always considered miracles as imaginary tales, fraudulent manipulations of real events or manifest symptoms of paranoia. So when I was faced with unplanned recoveries from incurable diseases, my scientific mind justified them by incomplete and commonplace answers such as, human biology has not yet been fully explored. Today I recognize the futility of this answer!

I remember the case of a young woman with a malignant brain tumor. I had removed it but had given her just a few months to live. Years later, she came back for a checkup and was found to be in good health. Her fiancée, a Sai Baba devotee, had taken her to India to see Sai Baba. After she left, we looked again at her medical records, and there was no doubt in our minds that it had been a case of terminal cancer. We were, naturally, quite skeptical and decided to classify this case as another unexplained recovery.

I now see the limitation of science which does not even try to explain the meaning of life or its significance to man. Our objective should be to realize the divinity inherent in each of us so that we may perceive what is incomprehensible both to man and science.

Before coming to Baba, I was unable to offer spiritual encouragement to my patients. Today, with my faith in Baba, and this spiritual consciousness, everything has changed. The spirituality that is now associated with my work helps me to recognize that the patient facing me, even though different in appearance, is divine just like me. I also realize that true service, accomplished with love and awareness, is a divine element. Sometimes, devotees of Sai Baba come to ask for a medical opinion. If I am faced with a difficult case, I recommend that they surrender to Baba who, at times, has performed miracles, but who always gives serenity when needed. I also encourage them to practice His teachings.

As you can see, meeting Baba has changed my vision of life. Not only has my approach to the medical profession changed but also the way I relate to people. Most dramatically, my approach to God has changed. Awareness of our inherent divinity and communion with the divine, as Baba recommends, helps us to become contented and grateful for whatever we receive and to realize the illusion of the phenomenal world in which we live.

Though I am now retired, I am still partly active in the medical profession. The rest of the time is spent working as a volunteer with Francesco and Paola on an *Education in Human Values* program that is in a number of public schools in Italy. During a recent interview with Baba, Francesco received confirmation from Baba that He fully approved his involvement in teaching human values in Italian schools.

Recently, I was in Venice for a teacher's seminar. We took the ferry to join another group of teachers. All of a sudden, I noticed a magnificent sailing boat with two huge masts. It was a beautiful sight, and I gazed at it until it disappeared from my view. At the close of the seminar, Francesco brought up the topic of the goal of existence. There was a long silence. It was obvious that the teachers were not used to discussing such a subject. To draw them out, and to skillfully avoid the sensitive topic of inner divinity, Francesco gave them some hints saying, it could be to become wiser, or to 'be' versus 'to have,' or to reawaken human values inside each of us. I suddenly felt the urge to say something. I told them, "Today, while coming here, I saw a marvelous sailing boat. Three years ago, all I wanted to do was to buy such a boat and spend most of my time on it. But today the goal of my existence has changed. Now all I want to do is to help and serve others."

So now I spend most of my time running from one school in the north of Italy to another in the south of Italy to help bring human values to our younger generation. This service has given me contentment and a wonderful sense of fulfillment. As Baba says, *Only through love can we have the vision of God.*

Walking With Baba
Ellyn Shander, M.D.

Medicine is my third profession. Sometimes it feels like I have had three lifetimes in one. When I was in my teens, I was a professional ballet dancer. At the old age of 20, I had to retire due to an injury. I then worked in the airlines for a few years, traveling for free to different parts of the globe. It was fascinating to travel, but I soon got bored with time schedules and the lack of challenges. I looked around at my life with discontent.

Ever since I was little, I have sought God, yet here I was with a feeling of emptiness and little purpose to my life. I had not yet gone to college and so, at the age of 23, I decided to tackle college, first at night and then full time. I eventually chose to go to medical school with the secret desire to be a psychiatrist. I say secret, because then, and still now, it is not fashionable to state that goal; it is much better to say you want to be a surgeon or a family practitioner.

I became a psychiatrist and have been in practice for 17 years, which has been an amazing time for me. In the early years of practice, I felt awkward trying to find the right words and to give the correct treatments but, over time, I have felt blessed every day by having the opportunity to help others and to grow myself. I know that the biggest change in me is how I now see my patients. Our improved healing relationship is a direct result of my studying and trying to embody the teachings of Sai Baba.

As I mentioned earlier, I have always sought a relationship with God, as well as divine answers that would make sense of this world. I remember rocking on my bed when I was about four years old and, in my mind, flying around the neighborhood looking down on all the houses. I would ask myself, "What was I supposed to remember? What was the reason that I chose this family and not those others? Why am I here?" I couldn't figure it out, and I was left with a nagging feeling that the answer was extremely important to me. Through the years I forgot the reason behind my search, but I always looked for God in synagogues, secret talks with angels, and ardent prayers to be successful. I was deeply disturbed by the Holocaust, frightened that the Nazis would return in the middle of the night. All through this time, I was searching for answers. I eventually lived in Israel, danced there, married there, and then returned to the United States. After one beautiful son, whose mission I know is to teach me patience and humility, I settled into practicing psychiatry.

Life seemed predictable then. I worked hard, tried to be a mom, weathered a divorce, and struggled to be a good doctor. But, one day, my life was dramatically altered.

A patient came to me with a horrific story of extreme child abuse at the hands of her family who believed in Satan. I listened with sadness and despair. I couldn't understand how anyone could harm one of God's children so horrifically. I did help her to leave her family and to try to attain some stability in her life. It was then that she told me that they now wanted to kill me.

I was frightened to "death." I bought big dogs for my home. I put in a new security system and, after going to gun school, I obtained a pistol with a permit. I spent months afraid and depressed. Suddenly one morning I woke up with a novel thought: "I don't want to live like this." Another thought kept running through my mind. "The opposite of fear is faith... Go look for God!" I don't know to this day where that thought came from, but it certainly changed my life. I decided that morning to start a journey to look for God again. I wanted to enjoy the sun and the flowers without being afraid, and what better place to start than in Jerusalem?

That very week I left alone on a trip to Israel and visited again the sacred sites that had always given me strength. I met beautiful people along the way, Christians and Jews, who shared with me their faith and love for God. I will never forget a small Jewish shopkeeper in Jerusalem who said to me, after hearing my request to buy a "powerful amulet" to keep away evil, "My child, all you need is faith. That will keep you safe." I smiled and knew he was right.

Later I made other trips. I visited a lovely ashram of devotees of Yogananda in California. I was invited to the Vatican for a fact-finding mission on child abuse. In Connecticut, I struck up a wonderful friendship with a Catholic priest who is now a close friend. All during my travels, people showed me how to live in faith, and my fear melted away. Then one day at a spiritual conference in Arizona, I saw a slide show on Sathya Sai Baba. I sat amazed as He gracefully walked amongst His devotees, and I immediately knew I wanted to meet Him. Little did I know that I was in for another major revolution in my life.

I have always lived my life with intensity, and so it was not surprising that I was on a plane for India within the month. I had heard that Baba had this gray substance with healing properties, and I wanted some for my mom, who lay dying in New York. If I had known then what I know now about Sai Baba, I wouldn't have been so arrogant. I bought bags of vibhuti in the ashram shop and presented them to Him at each darshan with a feeling of entitlement. I sat in the front row for almost every darshan in Brindavan, and I couldn't understand why Baba looked at me so fiercely and wouldn't stop to bless the vibhuti. After all, I was a doctor; I needed this stuff to be blessed for my patients!

Each day He would pass me with what I felt was disdain, and each day I would put away one more packet and present to him less vibhuti. On the last day, I just looked at him as He passed by and gave me a piercing look. I did not understand the significance of His divinity. I just felt morose at returning to New York without vibhuti for my mom. At the end of darshan, a small, beautiful, older Indian woman turned to me and said, "Swami knows what to give, and when." She then opened her pocket and gave me a small packet of vibhuti that she had received directly from Baba. She said, "Take this; it is special for healing." I burst into tears at her kindness. This was my first lesson from Baba of how He gives us gifts through others. It is through the compassion of other human beings that we can feel closest to Him.

I wanted to do something for Baba and the ashram. It has always been my way to "take on projects." On the way home in the plane, I fantasized about how I could volunteer to do something in India. I wanted to be important in Baba's eyes. I fell deeply asleep on the plane and had a dream: The roof of the temple at the ashram was leaking. Everyone was running over with ladders to try and fix it. I ran over with a ladder too. Baba stopped me and said, " No, you go home and fix your own roof first." I woke up embarrassed at my need for self-importance. But I got the message. I went home to study Sai Baba's message and to work on my own life.

Over the next few months, I read many books about Sai Baba. I especially loved *Sai Baba: The Holy Man and the Psychiatrist,* as it answered many of my questions about science versus faith. I called and found the Sai center in Norwalk, Connecticut, near where I live. This center has been my solace and source of learning and joy about Sai Baba. They have shown me patience when I have been ignorant and friendship when I have needed connection.

These have been extraordinary times. I met Sai Baba in August 1995, but it seems like centuries that we have known each other. I go to sleep thinking about Him, His pictures are all over my house, and daily I try to breathe and live His essence of love and compassion.

During the last four years since coming to Baba, my psychiatric practice has become more spiritual. I still dispense medication when needed, and I utilize many different therapy techniques, but I also speak about God and faith with almost every patient. My favorite question to ask them is, "Do you have a relationship with God?" I have gotten so many incredible answers. One patient has a beautiful personal relationship with God and reads the Bible daily. This has given her solace and comfort since her husband died. Sometimes she shares the scriptures with me. I then can share this knowledge with other patients when it is appropriate. One day, a young girl looked at me and said, "God is my higher power, and He protects me; actually, sometimes He is in my sneakers. They get me to an Alcoholics Anonymous meeting when I need to get there."

Some of my patients have described the presence of an angel or a guide that has been with them since childhood, protecting them. Of course, some of my patients don't have any relationship with God at all. One very depressed and suicidal young man spent hours trying to tell me that there was no God, just science. He could find no reason to live and struggled daily with feeling that there was no purpose to life. His hero, however, was Gandhi, and so I offered him books about Hinduism and Buddhism, which stimulated him intellectually. Slowly, he began to consider the possibility of a presence greater than himself. Today he is less depressed and not suicidal.

My patients give me the opportunity to experience an important lesson of Sai Baba's. Healing happens in the relationship between the healer and the patient through love and compassion. I have learned that keeping my heart open to each person that comes to me with their tears, despair, hopes, and complaints, strengthens my ability to be compassionate. I have expanded my practice to include patients with cancer and AIDS. It is through giving them hope, speaking about faith, and working on healing meditations, that I feel Baba intensely.

For instance, when I work with patients with cancer, I do guided meditations with music. With their eyes closed, I guide them to a sacred forest where they may see a spiritual being that will help them heal. I use the image of the sun to bring golden light into their bodies to heal every cell and every organ. I concentrate on every part of their bodies, thanking each limb and organ for doing its job. I remind them of wellness and, most of all, I bring the sensation of love into their consciousness. I do this by asking them to remember how it felt to hold a kitten or a puppy or a small baby in their arms. I ask them to allow this feeling of pure love and innocence to fill their bodies and flow throughout their being. It is at this moment that Baba really fills the office. Before I met Him, I wouldn't have had the courage to speak so openly about the healing miracle of love. Now I know that it is the most powerful healing force known. One of my patient's blood counts went up with the "good" white cells every time she listened to the meditation tape in the hospital as she recovered from cancer. While I create these meditations with my patients, an intimate relationship grows between us. I believe in their healing, and they feel my commitment. It is in this relationship that healing happens. I bring them hope until they can feel it for themselves. This is the gift Baba has given me in my life as well. When I am despondent or frightened, I remember that if Baba can love me and believe in me, then I can believe in myself. In my darkest moments, His words come to me: *When the night grows chill, don't you draw the blanket closer to you? So, when grief assails you, draw the warmth of the name of the Lord closer around your mind.*

In my office, I have a picture of Baba facing me; another one is by my seat. My patients cannot see these pictures, but I know His presence is pervasive. When I become impatient, I silently ask him for the patience to stay grounded, with my heart open. Baba has said, *Patience is all the strength a man needs.* If I am willing to listen to Him, I become more centered. If I am distracted by phone messages that require a response, or errands that I need to run, I try to breathe in Baba's energy and feel Him sitting in one of the chairs. When I feel nourished or held by Him, I can then nourish and be patient with others. Sometimes it is a matter of being quiet and waiting to see what happens after I have asked Baba for an intervention.

I remember sitting with one young girl who was obsessing about her weight and her anorexia for the hundredth time, despite many attempts on my part to redirect her. I felt my irritations grow, and I wanted to snap at her with annoyance. Looking at Baba's picture, without her noticing, I began to chant silently, over and over, "Om Namah Shivaya." After a short time, she began to cry quite intensely and speak about her loneliness. She had no friends and was not confident. When she began to cry, my heart melted and my annoyance disappeared. We started to talk about her despair at not being connected to anyone. Later in that session, she felt more hopeful about a social plan that we had worked on, and more confident with me. It was a turning point in her treatment. We also discovered that she loved butterflies, and now she reports that she sees them whenever she is lonely and asks God for help.

I try not to have preconceived ideas about my patients. I try to see each of them as an unfolding mystery. In medical school we are taught to have all the answers and to fix things, but I have learned from Baba that each person is a mysterious, unique creation. I sit and listen, asking Baba to reveal the mystery of this person to me. With His presence in the room, I have learned to feel safe in the unknowing. It is in this unknowing that the clues and hearts and souls of my patients emerge. For example, one day as I listened to a patient cry in despair about her childhood, I wondered silently how she was ever going to find her inner strength. In my mind I asked Baba for help. The patient suddenly looked up at me and told me a beautiful memory of how, when she was little, she used to hide in her local church and pray to the Virgin Mary. She had not remembered this for years. It began a life change for her. She brought Mary back into her life, and in our sessions she brings Mary's essence to both of us. Today her faith is strong, and she has begun the difficult task of recovering from incest.

At times, my patients tell me about their anger. When it is appropriate, I remind them of the need for righteous anger. Jesus threw out the moneychangers from his "Father's place" in righteous anger, and so we must know how constructive it can be when it involves protecting integrity. But at other times, they are spewing outrage and hate for others. I have heard disparaging comments made about gays, minorities, bosses, women, and people in politics. Or comments such as, "ethics and business don't mix." These are times that I actually feel pain in my heart for them. I can't always comment, so I pray silently and ask Baba to help them. I ask Him to open their hearts. Sometimes I imagine a golden triangle of light coming down over them from Baba, beckoning their highest potential to come forth. At these times, I feel a sense of relief. I know that Baba can handle the hate and negativity. This allows me to stay in the room without condemning the patient. If the person does not change at that moment, he or she at least has had an experience of their highest good being called upon. I do believe that Baba is the best co-therapist. We only have to remember to dedicate the work and the fruits of our labor to Him.

I treat many victims of child abuse in my practice. Their stories are very painful to me. I cry inside at the plight of the helpless child. In my mind, I ask Baba for the strength to listen; I ask Him to help this soul get strong. I also ask Him for help with my anger at the people who have perpetrated these crimes. I ask Baba to help me with my righteous anger, as I would like to see these people suffer for their crimes. But Baba has said to leave the evil to Him, and I try to remember His words as I work with my patients. *Whatever we do reacts upon us. If we do good, we shall have happiness, and if evil, unhappiness... People make their own palaces and their own chains and their own prisons.*

I have told my suffering patients that it is our spiritual challenge to rise above the bad acts that are done to us. I tell them to never let anyone's actions force them to close their hearts, and to walk their destiny with dignity, self-love, and compassion. In addition, in life we are given obstacles to overcome to make spiritual muscles. I find that when people are given a spiritual map that makes sense, it is both comforting and exhilarating.

Another part of creating that map in our lives involves visualizing and asking for what we want. Baba says we manifest our reality by our thoughts, words, and deeds. I ask patients to verbalize and visualize with me exactly what they want for their families and themselves. For instance, if someone wants a mate, I ask him or her to state out loud all the qualities that they want in a new friend. After good looking and other superficial items, people are usually able to articulate wanting qualities such as sensitivity, spirituality, and kindness in a potential relationship. I explain that we attract what we embody, which leads us to discuss how they can manifest these qualities in themselves. In addition, I ask them to change their language. For instance, someone might say, "I am always so lonely." I ask them to say, "I used to be so lonely, but now I am working on it." I have seen incredible changes in people as they begin to change their attitudes toward themselves and others.

Not coincidentally, when I am working on something very important to my own spiritual growth, a patient will appear who needs exactly the lesson that I am trying to learn. For instance,

Baba teaches that if you really walk in faith with Him, there is no fear. He says, *Faith in God is the toughest shield against the thrusts of fate.*

I have really tried to embody this principle. For years I have had a fear of walking outside at night. I have run like crazy from the car to the house, reliving my childhood fears of monsters and crocodiles. Since I have been with Baba, I have said to myself that faith is like pregnancy: you are either pregnant or you're not. You either walk in faith or not. In fact, it is impossible to be in fear and have faith at the same time; they are mutually exclusive. I explain that FEAR is an acronym; it stands for False Evidence Appearing Real. And I help people in whatever faith paradigm they feel comfortable with. I tell them to talk to God, make Him or Her real, ask for protection and comfort, and really walk in faith. I have learned from Baba that all roads lead to God. He says to respect every religion and path to God. Helping each person who comes to see me find their own relationship with God, the Great Transparency, Light Beings, or whatever they want to call this universal energy, has been the greatest blessing for me. By the way, I can now walk from the car to the house at a reasonable rate of speed, if I sing bhajans.

I have used Baba's teachings to help many people with anxiety, depression, and serious illnesses. Baba says that not a blade of grass moves on this earth without God's permission. I explain to my patients that we each have a journey to walk. How we react to life's events determines our destiny. A crippled person can react by spending their life bitter and feeling gypped. Or the same person can train for the Special Olympics. Often, illness is our greatest teacher. My patients that are recovering from cancer are reevaluating their professions and their attitudes about life. They are learning to love themselves and to change their priorities. I treat a woman now who has been cancer-free for one year after breast cancer and chemotherapy. She was a high-powered real-estate agent prior to her diagnosis. She hated the profession but was afraid to change jobs. During her illness we had many talks about how this cancer could bring about major spiritual and emotional changes in her life. Recovering from the chemotherapy taught her to be still and stop her frenetic activities. Talking to God, and walking in faith when she got scared, transformed her. She has gone from being a person who didn't often think about God, except for major holidays, to becoming a deeply spiritual person. Her new profession is creating sacred gardens for reading and meditation. They are magnificent. It has been a blessing for me to see her laughter and health as she discusses these projects.

Baba also teaches us to be happy and not to get caught up with maya, or the illusions of the world. So often people get depressed and anxious about their lack of material things, or how they look. He says, *Life is only the memory of a dream. It comes from no visible rain. It falls into no recognizable sea. Someday, not for a while yet, you will understand how meaningless it is to spend your whole life trying to accumulate material things.* I ask my patients to focus on their abundance, not their deprivations. With this in mind, I ask them to consider doing service for others. Baba often says that when we do service, it has far-reaching benefits for our own growth. Doing one nice thing for someone else every day goes a long way toward getting people out of their self-absorption.

Another major lesson that I am trying to embody is to see every person as the embodiment of God - to really see that we are the same, to see every human being that we meet as no different from us. I work each day on decreasing my judgments of others. I am usually in a hurry, and I become impatient with salespeople who keep me waiting. I often begin to get annoyed and disdainful. If I can catch my reaction quickly, I remember that this person is also God, just in a different costume. I try to say something appreciative and, invariably, I feel much better. I also try not to be critical or to gossip. In the hospital where I work in the mornings, people are always complaining and talking about the other staff members. I consciously try to walk into the hospital with Baba. Often I am singing bhajans in my mind or under my breath. When I decide to focus on feeling Baba with me, I don't participate in the complaining. Some days I am a dismal failure; other days I can see some headway. I do know that the longer I work on being a better person, the easier it is to notice when I need to correct myself.

I know that I am blessed with the best job on earth, because in order for me really to be a good healer, I must see each of my patients not only without judgment, but also as aspects of divinity. In other words, if I try to do my healing well, it requires me to work on being a better human being. Someone up there must have thought I needed a lot of help to put me in this position, but I love it! Baba teaches us to see others with compassion; I deeply appreciate the opportunity to work on this. I still get angry, annoyed, impatient, and tired. I try to remember that Baba is in the room with me. At those times, I look at His picture looking at me, sigh, and say to myself, "Yes Baba, I can do better."

The best gift has been when patients who have not seen me in years come to see me again and comment on how I have changed. They say I am gentler and kinder. I do hope that is true.

Walking with an avatar brings great responsibilities. It requires each of us to earn the title of devotee. I feel blessed to be given the opportunity to be a doctor and walk with Baba. Living up to His ideals of doing good, and doing no harm to others, is a responsibility each of us must take seriously. I recently had a dream after being very distressed about the news on television: I walked into a room and saw Baba standing there. I knew that He was God, and I was quite humble. I asked Him if I could put my forehead on His feet, and He consented. As soon as I put my head down, I began seeing horrible, violent pictures. I saw people in Tibet getting their skulls crushed, others being shot, people from all over the world being murdered. I cried and said, "Baba, when is it going to stop?" He answered with my exact words, "When is it going to stop?" I repeated my question, as I thought He didn't understand me. (My arrogance again; God not understanding me? Yeah, right.) He repeated it again, with great seriousness, "When is it going to stop?" At that moment, I understood His point. I remembered what Swami said, *The discontentment and disharmony in one's own self gets projected outside as chaos. Set your own Self in order, and you will find everything outside in order.*

The violence in the world will stop when each of us takes responsibility to stop the anger, criticisms, and negativity that we harbor in ourselves. We cannot say that the problem is outside of us across the world. We need to work on ourselves first.

I woke up with a serious thought. My working on myself might change the world just a little. But, maybe, if we all did it together, miracles could happen. Baba gives us a vision of just that miracle - a world where we are all connected to one another with love and compassion. I am incredibly grateful to be part of it.

The Divine Physician
Ramachandiran Cooppan, M.D.

The small figure with the bushy black hair and orange robe, now seen daily in Puttaparthi, India, will soon become the most recognized individual on the planet as the next millennium unfolds. Bhagavan Sri Sathya Sai Baba, the avatar for this age, has been dispensing unending love, compassion and hope to millions of devotees all over the world since He declared His mission at age fourteen. He has built schools, colleges and a Super Specialty Hospital and has transformed the small hamlet of Puttaparthi into a major spiritual center.

I grew up in South Africa and attended medical school there. This was during the repressive apartheid era. I wanted to get out and see what other parts of the world were like. My wife, Sarojini, and our first daughter left for Australia in 1969, and our journey has since taken us to Canada and finally the USA. During this time, we had two more daughters, and my wife has always been a friend and spiritual seeker with me.

My association with this incarnation of divinity started in 1979 when our family heard about Him from our relatives in South Africa. I had joined the Joslin Diabetes Center in Boston as a senior physician after completing a fellowship at the clinic from 1975-1976. That year had exposed me to diabetes in a way that I had never before experienced. Not only did I learn about the disease and interact with hundreds of patients but, also, the commitment to excellence that Dr Elliott Joslin, the founder, had championed was clearly evident on a daily basis at the clinic. While the dedication and caring for both patients and staff was an important factor in my accepting the position, I was also attracted by the fact that this was a nonprofit organization. The doors of the Joslin Clinic were open to all patients in need irrespective of their financial status.

These two ideals were very important to me, and I was thrilled to find them strongly in place at the institution where I was planning to make my career. From those early days and to the present, we continue to give free care and incur financial losses. But our policy will never change. We rely on our practice revenue, grants, and donations to allow us to continue our work. Last year, 1998, the clinic celebrated its 100th anniversary with multiple activities including an international diabetes symposium which attracted many experts to Boston.

The work has always been challenging and hard, because we are dealing with a chronic disease for which there is no cure. In the 1970's, there were even questions about the usefulness of tight glucose control in diabetes. The Joslin physicians were strong proponents of tight control due, in large measure, to Dr Joslin's experience and beliefs. Later, studies would vindicate this position. These patients are very demanding and prone to many complications which result in loss of vision, renal failure and vascular disease. In addition, many of them have serious psychosocial problems that also have to be addressed. We are a tertiary medical center. Other physicians refer patients to us, because we specialize in diabetes and in complicated patient problems. We, therefore, see some of the most challenging patients and have to try to come up with some solution for their problems. Since we conduct clinical research projects, sometimes we can enroll some of these patients in a clinical trial with new treatments that may help. At other times, we have to carefully review the situation and then give an opinion. For many patients, we are the last hope that something can be done for them. This is a tremendous responsibility, and we are determined to do everything possible to try and help these patients. We have to be realistic in our approach and work within the limitations of our therapies and of our patients.

When I joined the staff, in order to help build my practice, I was given new patients and transfers. We also have an active teaching program for fellows and residents and are also required to teach medical students. I invariably drew much of this duty, as well as coverage call, because the senior doctors were entitled to more time off. In the midst of all this, I was also studying to take my subspecialty board examinations for the USA. These were long and difficult days, but I managed to get through them by continuing my meditation and constantly remembering the Hippocratic oath I took when I was graduated.

As I reflect on my nineteen-year relationship with Baba, I find it has influenced not only my personal life but also my practice of medicine. It was my good fortune to be working at an institution where service with compassion and caring was part of our daily activity. One thing that working with chronic disease teaches you is humility and to become friends with your patients. As physicians, we are trained in the science of medicine, but we practice the art of medicine. We deal with people and their illnesses that cause them fear, pain, depression and even anger and hostility. We rely on our own inner strength and will. That enables us to continue to do our duty, day after day. I felt very strongly that I had to be compassionate, caring and patient. This feeling came from within me. It was the reason I chose to become a doctor. As a young man and medical student, I read about the lives of great physicians like Sir William Osler, the Mayo brothers, and the dedication and courage of men like Mahatma Gandhi and Albert Schwietzer. They inspired me, and I longed to emulate them.

As the years have passed, I still have a very busy practice. In fact, my practice is one of the largest in the group. I still see many patients every day in the office as well as in the hospital. I am now very involved in our continuing medical educational program and continue to teach the fellows, residents and medical students. I also carry out clinical research studies. Our educational program has grown tremendously in the last five years. This has resulted in continued airplane travel within the US as well as overseas. We have conducted seminars in Brazil, Japan, India and South America. Currently, I am planning a diabetes foot care course for February 2000 to take place in Vietnam, if we can raise the funds for the project. My colleague and I feel very strongly that we have a responsibility to go to this part of the world and help, especially after the terrible war that took place. We view these educational efforts as part of our mission, not only to do research in diabetes but also to treat the disease and help educate others in our treatment methods. We share our knowledge freely and readily, because it is the patients who will ultimately benefit by having better treatment.

I met Bhagavan Baba in December 1980 when my wife and I decided to go to see Him. It was soon after our family was introduced to Him by our relatives in South Africa. My parents had gone earlier and come back captivated by the avatar of the age. The memory of that first sight of Him is still alive in me today. I felt a strong attraction to Him because of the waves of love He emanates. There was no need for words. I saw and felt something deep inside me. This was my first impression of Baba. He was love incarnate and, over the years, it remains the strongest feeling I have.

We were very fortunate to be called in for an interview along with a group of South Africans. I was already caught up in the interview craze that permeates the ashram so, as I sat on the verandah, I could hardly believe this was happening. I had my first close glimpse of Swami that day. He looked at me sitting there and smiled. I was in heaven. We went in for the interview, and this moment remains one of the most precious experiences I have ever had in my life. It was here, in front of everyone, that Baba called me to sit at His feet and said. *He is doing my work.* I have held on to these words ever since. Whenever I am tired and find it hard to continue with my hectic work or travel schedule, I remember those words. When I cannot find enough time to participate in other service activities at our center and feel guilty about it, I remember Baba's words to me. I am doing His work, so I take courage and try to do more and ask Him for strength. In the past nineteen years, that was the only time I have spoken with Baba or kissed His feet; but the feelings and deep emotions it generated have stayed with me and have only become stronger with time. Swami is an ocean of love. We are droplets of love. When our love meets, they merge, and this binds us to Him and allows Him to slowly transform us.

As a physician, it is natural for me to be focussed on Baba as the ultimate physician, all knowing and all-powerful. His life has been His message, and He asks that our life becomes an example too. Swami is a physician who never stops giving and helping, day in and day out, listening to all our concerns and worries petty as they are. He is there for us, giving of Himself selflessly and lovingly for all these years. This is not just another holy man.

Only one who is Self-realized and in total control of all the senses can function with this degree of intensity for so long.

After coming back from seeing Baba, I did not immediately notice any dramatic changes at work. Working in a group practice, where I was the only Indian, I was not ready to say too much to my colleagues about this experience. Some of them noticed the green ring Baba had made for me during the interview and were curious. I said it was a present from someone special and left it at that. This satisfied most, until they walked into my office and saw a photograph of Baba. At that point I told them a few things about my visit and His teachings. No one asked me for a book to read, but they appeared to respect my belief as I did theirs. I noticed that my meditation was definitely different from earlier. I found I could meditate more easily and for longer periods of time. This has to be the effect of coming in contact with the avatar. I started to go to the Brookline Sai Center more regularly and began meeting other devotees and hearing their experiences. Regional meetings and retreats became a part of my life.

My workload increased even more, and I had many difficult patients who continued to need care. With this came more "on call" nights and weekends. Weekend call was very hard at the clinic, because the on call doctor took care of all patient phone calls. We can get up to 30-40 calls a day and at all hours of the day and night. We did not allow our fellows in training to do this part of the work, because we felt it was the senior doctors' responsibility to take care of emergencies and advise patients on the phone. In addition, you went to the hospital to do rounds, and most of the patients were very sick. It is not unusual for us to get phone calls from people who were not even our patients but who had called because someone had told them about us. In these cases, I tell myself that these people are frightened and in pain and they need help. So we not only listen to them but suggest a course of action whenever possible.

As hard as the days were, I was starting to notice that I was more at ease with my practice, except when I was on call duty. This I did, gritting my teeth. I found that I looked forward to seeing my patients, not out of a sense of obligation or because they were paying for the visit, but because this was the right thing to do. These people were ill and needed help, and I wanted to help them. I really started to help them, not as a duty, but because we were all connected to each other. Somehow, meeting Baba created this feeling in me. When I connected to Him, I in fact, was connecting to all. I also found that my efficiency was improving. I found that I could increase my productivity when the need arose. I had always been someone who worked well, but I now noticed that my intuition was sharper and that many coincidences were happening. For instance, if I needed to meet a colleague to discuss a patient, I would run into the person in the hospital corridor, or the person would call my office later that day. Soon, I came to realize that this was not coincidence but the working of His divine hand in helping to make things happen when the service was for the greater good.

The area where I noticed the most change was in dealing with my patients and their problems. I was becoming a better listener and was giving them more time to speak with me about their concerns. I remember a particularly difficult patient whom I had to care for before I met Baba. This person tested my courage and resolve to its limits. He had painful diabetic neuropathy, was addicted to narcotics, and had a personality problem as well. He was abusive and demanding and called the office so much that it was disruptive. His demands for narcotics lead him to many hospitals and emergency rooms in the city; and invariably, I was called about him. The problems escalated. He called me at home at all odd times. I was even visited by the federal narcotics agency because of his heavy drug use. No other physician would take over his care, and I struggled to keep my balance taking care of him. It seemed that I was stuck with this man. I knew the only way to deal with this case was to take one day at a time. This patient continued to test me; but after meeting Baba, I tried to not react to his tirades the way I had before. I just did my duty and left the rest to Swami. This was at a time when there was starting to be pressure to increase the number of patients each doctor saw in a day. This was not only in our clinic but with doctors everywhere.

Another change that I see now is that when a patient is late, I no longer become irritated, because this can be a problem at the end of a long and busy day. If I am running late with my program, I go to the waiting room and inform my patients about this. The fact that I take the time to talk to them has made a great difference. When they see me later, they are calmer and more understanding. I have seen Baba minister to all the devotees who come to Him over the years and at no time is He upset, curt or angry. He continues to pour out His love and compassion and listen to all, taking letters, smiling and just being there. This is the divine physician at work, and I try to remember that constantly, and it makes me feel stronger. Now when I start to examine a patient, I pray to Baba to guide and help me.

I have also found that the breathing of my patients, as I listen to their lungs, is saying, "so hum" to me all the time. Knowing Baba, I appreciate the enormous significance of this. I am constantly being reminded that HE and I and WE are One. As medical students, we are taught very early on to listen to the patients breathing as part of the physical examination. With a stethoscope, we listen to the movement of the air in and out and can detect disease states from the alterations in the quality of this process. With breathing in, air enters the lungs and has a "sho" quality to it, and with breathing out, it has a "humm" quality. These are normal respiratory sounds to us, and we listen in a routine way, paying attention to changes that may be present. If we detect no abnormalities, we say the breath sounds are normal. After meeting Baba, I read His explanation of meditation and the movement of air in and out of the lungs. It was here I learned about "So Hum." I cannot remember exactly when this light went off in my head. It was around the time when I started praying to Swami before touching my patients, when I started to examine my patients in a more reverential frame of mind. I start with a brief prayer to Baba to work through me and for Him to ease the pain of the patient. It was not any sudden revelation when I realized the significance of the breathing process; it grew with time and appeared as something natural. It was Baba opening up my awareness to what was going on all the time. He was reminding me of a great truth that I could carry with me in my daily role as a physician. As I reflect on this now, I can appreciate how all of nature is constantly reminding us of this basic message of unity. All we need to do is to open up our hearts and minds to this truth. The key to unlocking this door is to act with love and to be caring.

I also notice that when the end of the day approaches and I am tired and yet another patient has to be seen, I no longer look at this as a burden but tell myself that I have another opportunity to be of service to someone in need. Thinking about what Baba would want me to do in these situations helps me to arrive at this state of mind. If I am really tired, I quickly go to my office and close my eyes and pray for strength. There is a picture of Baba on my desk next to the phone. It serves to remind me to speak kindly to the other person at all times, even though there are times when it is my inclination to slam down the phone.

I have always tried to be friends with most of my patients. Sometimes, when one of them dies, I feel as if I have failed him. I would constantly review things to make sure something was not missed that could have saved his life. As an example, when a patient is in the intensive care unit there are many consultants called in. As the primary physician in charge of the patient, I read all the notes, review the laboratory tests, and speak to the residents and others to make sure we are all communicating with each other and have a common goal. This is a very time consuming task; but it needs to be done, and someone has to take the responsibility to do it. As the internist, I take on this role for my patients in the hospital. When this is done, and the family is kept informed of all the events, then even a poor outcome is accepted.

Growing up in an Indian home and family, I was aware of the principle of karma and the teaching of the immortality of the soul. But this was an abstract understanding. I did not feel it to be real, nor had I met anyone who, I felt, really understood and lived this belief. That was until I met Bhagavan Baba. *My Life is my Message, Help ever, Hurt never,* these were statements that Baba made, and it was evident to all who wanted to see that it was the truth. Baba has made spirituality come alive for me. I have seen

Him and experienced His love, and I know that He is an embodiment of the divine who is here to guide and teach us.

This experiencing of the Sai phenomenon has slowly become part of my daily practice. I have heard the avatar speak and reiterate the ancient knowledge, and I know that I cannot control death. It is mind boggling that this is Rama, Krishna, Jesus and Buddha come again to show us the way. Even as a physician, my skill and knowledge comes from God, and my duty is to do the best I can and leave the rest to the Lord. I do this now not from a sense of resignation to the inevitable but, rather, with the conviction that whatever I do matters if it is done with love and caring.

I now try to be with some of my patients when they die in the hospital, and I pray with the family at the end. I feel more comfortable than ever speaking to them about a loving and caring God. I express my belief in our oneness more openly. This I attribute mainly to my experience with Baba. His language of love has opened the hearts of my patients. I remember one older patient of mine who always used to bring me articles on health and vitamins. He took many supplements daily. However, he landed in the hospital desperately ill and was dying. I called his wife to meet me that afternoon. We both stood by his bed and prayed for him, and I was there as he took his last breath. There was a quiet calm in the room. I looked at the wife, and she had tears in her eyes. She thanked me for being her husband's doctor and his friend. I reminded her of the many times when her husband and I had talked about life and death and about God. We spoke about how her husband was always smiling and loving. Even before the critical turn in events in the hospital, he and I spoke of praying and asking for God's help in our times of need. Because we had set the stage earlier in our relationship, I felt at ease talking with his wife in this way. She hugged me. We parted with no more words, but her face was filled with love. Moments like these are rare. They serve to remind us of the need to cultivate the trust and love of our patients. Without this, we lose one of the most important things we do as doctors. Not only must we know how to cure illness but, also, we need to know how to counsel our patients about the end of earthly life. This need not be left only to our colleagues from the different religious groups who work with us; we too need to feel comfortable with this role.

Even now, when I meet a difficult patient or have to give unpleasant news, I pray to Baba for strength and courage. I have found that when we are prepared to be humble and to be ourselves, forsaking the pull of the ego, we can then become instruments of the Lord. Our creative energy and love will flow and even the difficult and impossible situations can be managed with care and dignity. I was actually with the troublesome patient I mentioned when he passed away in a coma. This was many years after my meeting Baba. Many of my friends asked me if I felt a sense of relief. In one way I did. Our office phones no longer rang all the time, and staff no longer had to live in daily terror. But I also had a sense of sadness. This man was a good person who had a difficult disease. I am glad that I was able to live through this and be able to be of some service to him. I am sure that without Baba's help I would have become cynical and run the risk of abandoning my obligation as a physician.

Asking Baba for help is not a sign of weakness but an affirmation that the creator of All is indeed all-knowing and all-powerful. The dawn of truth comes when one realizes that the Baba we call on is also the Baba within us and in everyone and in everything. We know this to be true because Baba has told us it is so. But we need to experience and, from experiencing, know it is the truth. This is not easy, and I constantly ask Swami to help. Sometimes after meditation, I have this sense of oneness, but it does not last. I also have this experience when I am deeply engaged in helping a patient in need. The sense of calmness and love in these moments is unbelievable. There is no need for anything but to be available and to do whatever is needed. When the action springs from this basis, it is filled with energy and empathy and the Lord guides it.

A few years ago, I had the opportunity to consult on a young child from India with diabetes, whom the parents brought to our institution for treatment. After I examined the youngster, I invited the family to my office to discuss a few more issues. I stepped out for a moment and, on my return, the parents had a huge smile on their faces and said, "Sairam." They had seen Baba's photograph on my desk, and this made me very happy. Then, after I spent forty-five minutes talking with them and telling them that I felt that the little girl would need insulin for the rest of her life, the mother looked at me and said, "But Baba said the disease would go away." I was taken aback for a moment, and I saw they were waiting expectantly for me to say something. I looked at Swami's picture, took a deep breath, and then told them that I did not doubt the word of the avatar; but for now, she needed treatment with insulin. I knew that I was rendering the treatment she needed at the time and was happy to leave the future to Baba. Unfortunately, I never found out what eventually happened to her.

On another occasion, it was close to the end of a very busy day, my last patient was a little late, and I was just starting to fade a little. I actually was hoping that he would not show so that I could end the day. But then, my nurse called and said he had arrived. So I walked in trying to be cheerful, and this man smiled widely and said, "Sai Ram, Dr. Cooppan." It was as though I had been given a shot of adrenaline. I felt wonderful and ready to help him. In fact, the visit went longer than planned as we spoke about Baba as well as about his diabetes. I have reflected on this experience often, and I know that I may not see another patient who is a devotee for a long time. However, I have started to realize that all my patients were saying "Sai Ram" to me; it is just that I was not listening. I need to remember that every time one of them greets me, it has the same meaning. It comes from their hearts, and I must open mine to receive it. The best way is to be yourself, to smile and return the greeting with love and caring. This is what Baba teaches us over and over with his endless discourses and writings.

Today, there is a crisis in health care in the USA as well as in other parts of the world. The problem varies from lack of resources all the way to the impact of managed care. These are major issues that require all who are involved in health care policy and delivery to reexamine. We need to regard access to good timely care as a fundamental human right. Bhagavan Baba has also set the tone for medical care in the next millennium. He has established a Super Specialty Hospital in Puttaparthi. This magnificent structure was built in less than a year and gives free care to all in need. It offers the best modern treatment for cardiovascular problems as well as renal diseases. They do renal transplants and open heart surgery and have outstanding results with very low infection rates and short length of stay. All of the staff are devotees of Baba, and the place is more like a temple of healing than a hospital filled with modern technology. There is a quiet peace and calm throughout, and you can sense that this is a holy place. This hospital's care has been so outstanding that the government of Karnataka has donated land to Baba and requested Him to build another similar hospital in Bangalore. The providing of this type of specialized care for poor children and adults, who could never afford it, is indeed a gift from God. In addition, there is a general hospital in Puttaparthi that has served hundreds of locals for many years. During major festivals, when hundreds of thousands come to see Baba, the hospital gets additional help from visiting physicians and nurses.

In a recent discourse, Swami spoke about diabetes and clearly stated that the majority of adult diabetes was a life style issue with genetic factors being involved. He advised the doctors to work with the patients on proper nutrition and exercise to reduce the risks of complication. He even stated that in those with poor control, oral drug therapies were preferred to insulin. This latter statement reflects our recent under-standing of the basic role of insulin resistance in causing this type of adult onset diabetes. These lectures and insights serve to demonstrate to me the omniscience of Baba and His complete knowledge of all things. The following quotation illustrates the deep truth of His message, its simplicity and timelessness. *Moderation in food, moderation in talk and in desires and pursuits, contentment with what little can be got by honest labor, eagerness to serve and to impart joy to all, these are the most powerful of all tonics of health-preservers known to the science of health, the Sanathana Ayurveda. (Sadhana, the Inward Path p 170.)*

I now view each patient of mine as being referred to me by Bhagavan Himself. As a devotee of His, I endeavor to do my very best for each one of them, and I leave the rest to Swami. Today, I am starting to awaken to the enormous importance of the advent of the Sai avatar. His mission is the spiritual transformation of mankind, moving us to the next level of our destiny so that we will act and live as divinely inspired beings. This is the task this triple incarnation has taken on. There can be no greater undertaking on the planet for the future of mankind. As a physician, I am drawn naturally to His advise on health issues and find myself thanking Him for drawing me to Him and for giving me this opportunity to make this journey of discovery. Swami has said that the most important discovery during this life on earth is the inner journey towards the realization that we are divine, immortal beings. The result of this process, as it slowly unfolds, is that we act as divinely-inspired human beings. This means we need to emulate the way divinity reveals itself when it embodies in the human form. Bhagavan Baba is the supreme example of this. His life is one that is filled with loving, caring and giving.

I have come full circle now. Having spent the last twenty-five years at the Joslin Clinic, I find that I have become a chronic doctor for these chronic patients. I have seen them grow, marry, have families and live wonderfully productive lives. I have also seen them complete the cycle and pass on. In all of these years, my patients have been great teachers to me. They have shown me what courage is and what hope is all about, and they have also reminded me daily that my present good health is to be used unsparingly for helping them and others.

My colleagues now know a little about Baba and where I go in India. Most know that I spend twenty-four hours chanting for world peace during the akanda bhajan and make sure I am not on call at the time. I, myself, feel more comfortable talking about Swami. Some of my patients have asked for books, and one even went to a Sai center. I now travel quite extensively as the assistant director of our educational programs. Every time I give a lecture, I pray to Baba and thank Him for using me to help spread our expertise and knowledge of diabetes to others. I view this as an extension of my duty to *help ever, hurt never*. Every now and then, when I least expect it, a physician comes up to me after the lecture and says "Sai Ram." So, His devotees are all around and listening.

Baba has become a part of everything I know and do. The next step for me is to work on myself to continue to grow spiritually. I need to deepen myself by being more regular with my meditation, to reflect more on what I read from Baba and not just collect information. I like to read and am always thrilled by someone who writes in a way that makes me sit back and ask questions. I am always attracted to those who write about the relationship between science and spirituality. Inevitably, both science and spirituality come back to the same place, completing the circle from emergence to merging.

This reflecting and reassessing is fundamental for making progress in life. I want to experience that sense of oneness, not only sporadically but throughout most of the working day. The love, the deep sense of calm, and the energy that this state brings make everything we do so special. There is no need for anything else but the joy that comes from being alive and aware. I know where I need to look for the answer, for Swami has said that mankind suffers from physical illness as well as spiritual illness. His treatment for this is to cultivate virtue, for it cures both. To be of service to others is an opportunity to cultivate virtue. We should, therefore, welcome our patients as messengers of God, sent not only for their benefit but more for our own spiritual growth and progress. I, therefore, pray to Swami to be ever with me and to give me more opportunities to be of service.

Sai Baba and the Psychiatrist
Teerakiat Judo Jareonsettasin, M.D., M.R.C. Psych (U.K.)

Introduction to Sai
My journey to God started in 1980 when I was a first-year medical student. I was regularly attending Dr. Jumsai's lectures on spirituality, which were given in Bangkok at the Mind Club at Chulalongkorn University, where I studied medicine. At that time neither of us knew of Sai Baba, and I regarded Dr. Jumsai as my first spiritual teacher. However, later, Dr. Jumsai became a well-known and well-loved devotee of Sai Baba. When he presented Baba as God, I could not understand this and, therefore, stopped attending his lectures. However, in 1984, I returned to the club during my unhappiness over a conflict with my girlfriend. I was very sad then and, in an attempt to allay my own depression, I read the book *Sai Baba, The Holy Man and the Psychiatrist* by Dr. Samuel Sandweiss. After reading a few pages, I intuitively knew that Sai Baba was God. I wanted to see Him, and I finally arrived in Prasanthi Nilayam on Febuary 3, 1985. I was extremely fortunate to be called in for an interview the next day.

Encounter
Swami took me into the interview with another Thai lady and asked me to translate for her. He told the lady that she had had sinusitis for the last 25 years, and He had come to her in two dreams. She admitted that this was true. Certainly, a doctor would never say that to a patient! A few days later, I was called in again with a group of new devotees from Thailand. The men were waiting for Swami in front of His interview room on the veranda. I was sitting next to a Thai man who was extremely fat. It was his first visit, and he wanted Swami to help him with his health problems. He did not speak English and asked me in a whisper, while waiting for Swami to finish darshan, "Boy, do you speak English?"

"Yes," I replied.

"Can you tell Sai Baba that I have Bowwan and a leg problem? Do you think it should be called leg ache or leg pain?"

"Of course," I said, "Diabetes is the word for Bowwan, and leg pain sounds better to me."

Swami then came on to the veranda and ushered us into the interview room. He shut the door, went over to that man and asked, *Sir, how is your leg problem?* He paused a little and added, *and diabetes. Don't worry. I will take care.*

It is not difficult to imagine how excited that Thai man was when I translated what Swami had said to him. Unfortunately, I have never met that man again to find out the outcome.

Reflecting on these incidents, I was deeply touched by how intimate Swami was with us, knowing all our preoccupations and speaking to us at just the right moment. What a great physician He is! Gradually, over the years, I have become absorbed in His teachings and have tried to practice them as sincerely as possible. Swami told me to practice love and do all work as God's work. So, before I see a patient, I calm my mind and put out loving thoughts. It is very easy to do if I am not busy, but during critical times when there are many patients to see, a lot of administrative work to do, and the family to look after, the only thing that keeps me in balance is remembering Swami's sayings. Once Swami mocked me in an interview, saying that I always say, "Quick, quick." He warned me that I should not be in a hurry. He said, *Haste makes waste. Pregnancy takes nine months, but some people want the baby to be born quickly, which is impossible. Be patient.* I often get impatient and do things quickly, but Swami has slowed me down quite a lot.

I have had many interviews with Swami that confirmed His omniscience. One time, I was with a Thai lady in an interview. She had consulted me about possibly having heart disease. She was quite worried. When she asked Swami to help with her heart disease, Swami reassured her that she did not have any heart problem. Turning to me, He said, *How can she have a heart problem when I am here? She only has high cholesterol, no heart problem.*

After I became a doctor, I went for my postgraduate training in psychiatry and child psychiatry in London. Eventually, I obtained membership in the Royal College of Psychiatrists in the United Kingdom. I returned to Thailand to teach and practice in a semi-rural town in the northeast about 250 miles from Bangkok. I also have a private practice in Bangkok two weekends each month. Throughout these years, I have been very active in the Sai Organization. Once, I told Swami that I wanted to give up my private practice in order to have more time for His work. Swami, being very practical, told me not to do it, because I needed the money.

Basic Practice

I would like to share how Swami helps in my work. This has to do with a fundamental belief about human nature. The Western theories of psychology teach that we are no different from animals; we are actually a kind of animal. But Swami says we are no different from God; we are divine. Although Swami does say that, we all have animal qualities. He says this is not our basic nature. The western psychiatrists are not wrong, but they are not completely right either. The question is how do we reconcile these beliefs? Whether or not we are divine is not the issue. What we need to do is to take a belief that we sincerely hold and try to live that belief wholeheartedly. In my case, I try and live my life as if we are all God. To do this requires a conscious effort. If I forget or get upset about something, I remind myself that God is behind every event, even though sometimes it doesn't look that way.

It is not my job to convince anybody of this belief. I just listen to whatever theory they have and do not denigrate it; that does not mean I have to believe it. Swami says one has to be confident about one's own belief and experience but, at the same time, not disturb the faith of others. My colleagues know that I am a Sai devotee and, if they asked me about Sai, I would tell them. Though they do not share my view, they do not dislike me, and, in fact, they are curious about Swami. In this way, I believe that I represent Sai best by my example.

I try to see God as the basic nature in everyone. For example, I try to see Swami in every patient I work with. At the bodily and social levels, I treat patients according to their status and action. If patients become violent or uncontrollable, I may have to use drugs to calm them down, knowing full well that the medications are only for the body; the divine inside is intact and remains as witness. At the same time, I have the opportunity to practice that the God in me is the witness to everything that happens. Swami says that when we begin this practice it requires imagination but, that over time, it becomes a reality.

In clinical practice, seeing Sai in every patient and circumstance has taught me to be humble and calm and to trust that everything is done by God's will. I always do my best without telling the patient this, as I do not think it is either necessary or appropriate. I am playing my part in His play, the part of a good doctor that the patient can trust. Once, when I was quite new to psychiatry, I had a violent patient who threatened to kick me. He looked restless and aggressive. I was caught unprepared and did not know what to do or say. He was about to move toward me, but I suddenly remembered Swami and imagined myself sending the patient white light and love. Immediately, to the amazement of the nurses watching the whole scenario, he stopped and became relaxed. In order not to forget Swami, I often imagine Him in the consulting room with me, sitting in a vacant chair I keep for His imaginary presence. I imagine Him listening to the patient, and I mentally pray to Him to help me say the right thing.

One caution: some therapists like to talk about God to their unwilling patients. I believe it is usually a display of ego on their part, wanting to show the patient how spiritual he or she is, or how much God loves them. Perhaps, sometimes, the therapist even wants the patient to feel he or she has some special knowledge or secret.

Secret for Psychiatry

In psychiatry, we deal with the mind. Once I asked Swami, "How can we transform our mind?"

Swami replied, *It is very easy. Before you do anything or have any thought, think whether it is good or bad, right or wrong. This is called discrimination. There are two types of discrimination, individual and fundamental.*

"What is fundamental discrimination?" I asked.

Swami continued, *Fundamental discrimination is when you inquire whether what you do or think is good or right for everyone or not. Individual discrimination is often selfish, and you should follow fundamental discrimination.*

I was delighted to learn this secret about how we can transform our mind, and I have tried to apply it in my practice. In psychiatry we are taught to be non-judgmental, but this needs re-examining in the light of Swami's teachings. Those who proclaim that to be judgmental is bad are usually the most judgmental people. In fact, they rank non-judging as better than judging! Isn't that a form of judging? Once I saw a patient who told me he wanted to do all kinds of bad things to retaliate against his estranged wife. I could not sit still and be non-judgmental. I challenged his thoughts and asked him if what he was thinking was right for him. Of course, I did this after I had listened to everything the patient had to say. It worked. It doesn't mean that I am more righteous or that I know better. But we all know, deep inside, what is right and what is wrong. I am reminded of the advice Swami gave to a psychiatrist. He said the way to practice psychiatry was to listen patiently until he understood and felt the patient's life deeply. *Then, when you and the patient are one, you can teach him about our reality.*"(*Spirit and the Mind,* by Dr. Samuel Sandweiss p. 192)

The fact that you can examine your thoughts and make a judgment about whether your thoughts are good or bad, right or wrong means that you actually can step aside and watch your thoughts. In effect, you transcend the thoughts. You no longer identify yourself with your thoughts. You are above and beyond them. So who are you then? Inquire further and you will find out for yourself. It is so wonderful to learn this secret from the Lord Himself.

More Teachings on Psychiatry

How many kinds of knowledge are there? Swami asked me in an interview.

I ventured to answer: "Swami said five."

Good. What is the highest knowledge? Swami asked further.

"Practical knowledge."

Swami then said, *How do you get to practical knowledge?"*

"By putting Swami's teachings into practice," I replied.

Swami said, *No, not correct - only by discrimination knowledge. Discrimination knowledge leads to practical knowledge, and what comes before discrimination knowledge?*

Having just given the wrong answer, I kept quiet.

Swami then supplied the answer, *General knowledge comes before discrimination knowledge, and superficial knowledge before general knowledge, and bookish knowledge before superficial knowledge.* He then summarized, *Bookish knowledge leads to superficial knowledge, which leads to general knowledge, which leads to discrimination knowledge, which leads to practical knowledge.*

What a wonderful exposition on the different types of knowledge! I can relate this teaching to my early training in psychiatry. As a novice in the psychotherapy unit in a hospital in London, I was anxious about learning the techniques of psychoanalysis. I read a lot of books, attended all kinds of academic seminars on the subject, and had therapy myself. I felt quite confident when it was time to meet with a patient. After a few sessions, the patient confronted me, saying that I spoke as if my words came from a textbook. I was shocked. He was completely right, and I learned my lesson. In trying to interpret what the patient said, I quoted what I read from the textbook of psychotherapy or what my professor said in the supervision sessions. It did not come from practical knowledge of being with the patient and using my discrimination. Instead, I borrowed the knowledge from books or others. With experience, I have gradually gotten better. Now I bring more spontaneity to psychotherapy sessions, along with the added benefit of feeling the presence of Sai Baba.

Secret in Medicine

Recently Swami showed some of us a model of His new hospital in Bangalore. He said He would open the new hospital for three specialties: heart, kidney, and brain surgery. He said equipment (nowadays) was expensive, but He was not worried as he had good thoughts and money kept coming. He wanted His hospital to be clean and comfortable. I asked Him about heart transplants, and Swami replied, *Doctors do not tell you the result of the transplant after a few months. The result may be good on the first day, but not so good after that. After all, people do not give their heart when they are alive, but the heart has no use after their death.* He chuckled. Then He talked about a natural spare heart valve inside the heart and, in fact, said valvular heart patients do not need an artificial valve. When I asked Him to repeat this statement, He kindly agreed. But I still do not understand this, despite my medical background. He then added, *Doctors do not know this secret, but I know.*

Sai in Psychiatric Practice

I once asked, "How about psychiatry? Could Swami say something about psychiatry?" He smiled and said, *Imagination for both the patient and the psychiatrist. They talk....* After that, I could not follow what Swami said. In my practice of child psychiatry, I find that I rely on Swami's teachings on parenting more than any theory I have learned during my training. The balance between love and discipline is what I refer to most when I give advice to parents who come for consultation about problems with their children. I often tell the children in therapy stories that Swami tells in His discourses. Once I was on call at the emergency clinic. A young girl came to see me in a suicidal state. She felt hopeless and saw no way out of her problems. After listening to her, I offered to admit her to the hospital, which she refused. I didn't know what to do but felt the urge to tell her a story. I told her Swami's story of two frogs, one thin and the other fat, who fell into a bucket of milk. The fat frog gave up, sank, and died, but the thin frog kept on swimming until the milk turned to butter allowing it to jump out and survive. The patient's face lit up; she smiled, thanked me, and said that she had hope again. She asked me about the origin of the story, and I told her that my teacher had taught it to me.

Even Swami's specific teachings, such as the light meditation, can be applied in psychiatric practice with both adults and children. I once had to treat a very aggressive young man in London. Having failed in a few Western methods, I told the man, "Look, I come from the East. We believe in a natural method. When the sun rises, darkness just disappears, without the sun using any force. You are filled with a lot of anger and hatred. Shall I apply this principle of replacing darkness with light? Are you interested?" He agreed. I then led him in the light meditation that I had learned from Swami, spreading love to everyone at the end. After ten minutes, the patient opened his eyes, which were filled with tears. He said he had never felt like this before. He improved so much that, when I reported this treatment to my professor, I did so with trepidation, as I had used an unconventional method. He said, "I always prefer a positive method but do not know how to go about it. I have had to wait for 30 years for an Oriental student to tell me how." He was so pleased that he asked me to make an audiotape of the light meditation for the patients and staff of the unit in which I was working.

On one occasion, I had to present a paper on "Buddhism and Psychotherapy" to an academic audience at a university hospital in London. I explained the Buddha's core teaching on detachment, quoting the Buddha's saying, "Nothing in this world is worth clinging to." If we want to get rid of suffering, we have to be detached. One eminent psychoanalyst came to me after the talk and said that this was exactly the goal of genuine psychoanalysis. He became very interested in Buddhism afterward.

Detachment

Swami once came to me in a dream to teach me about detachment. He said, *Practice detachment.* I asked, "How, Swami?"

He then explained, *Detachment is deep attachment to God.*

Later, He came in another dream and said, *Attachment is detachment from God.*

I have had the opportunity to relate these dreams to devotees in the presence of Swami. He confirmed that He had taught me this in dreams, saying that I was right to say that the mind needs something to hang on to, and deep attachment to God is really true detachment from the world. In fact it is not difficult to practice detachment. We have to stop thinking the thoughts that bother us and replace them with other thoughts. Once I saw a patient who told me he didn't know what to do with his mind. He said he could not stop thinking and that even his thoughts gave him troubles. I treated him for a few months to no avail. One day I remembered Swami's teaching that the mind is like a television. I asked the patient, "If you do not like a particular program on the television, what do you do?" He responded, "Change the channel to a program I like better." In the same way, I told him, he should do this with his mind. It worked.

Swami says the mind needs something to hold on to, and that something should be God; otherwise, the mind will always move and jump about here and there like a mad monkey. He once said to a friend of mine in an interview, *The mind is always in motion, experiencing the emotion of commotion, promotion, and demotion; no devotion, devotion deep in the ocean!*

True Human

Swami says that a true human must have unity of thought, word, and deed. Now, I know that Swami has a program called Education in Human Values, but He also uses the term 3HV instead of EHV. I was puzzled by this and recently asked Him in an interview, "Swami, can you explain 3HV to me?"

He said that 3HV are the harmony of head, heart, and hand.

I was wondering about those who had unity of bad thoughts, bad words, and bad deeds! I asked Him, "Are they human?"

Swami replied, *There are such people in the world, and you should not pay attention to them.* He then explained that purity comes before unity, which will then lead to divinity. He said, *Without purity, there will be no unity, only community, no divinity.*

This has helped me understand that 3HV actually means not only unity, but also purity of thought, word, and deed. In fact it comes from the Sanskrit words *trikarana suddhi*. *Trikarana* means the three inner instruments of thought, word, and deed, and *suddhi* means purity.

Conclusion

I consider myself very lucky to have had the chance to be taught by Swami. I have tried to relate my experiences with Him and His teachings as objectively and truthfully as possible.

I have changed a lot since coming to Swami, and my wife and my mother can confirm this. I used to be very impatient, easily irritable, and very ambitious. Over the years I have become calmer and can let go of things more easily, to the point that my teachers in the UK could not believe what I used to be like. One psychiatrist friend of mine said, "You are so happy that whoever can irritate you must be really irritating." I regard this as a compliment for Swami. I tell my friends that this transformation is the result of having Swami as the teacher to guide me in life.

I think we need to humble ourselves in order to receive His blessings and, especially, His grace. We can see when Swami is not pleased with our ego. If we love Him, we would not do things that do not please Him. He teaches me that we can purify the mind by not acting in the wrong way.

There is no better time to live than now, when God is so near physically. Swami teaches us that there is only God, in all His or Her radiant wonder. All the good and the evil, the very best and the very worst, the virtuous and the devious, each and every one, are absolutely perfect manifestations of God as they are. May we all realize this truth.

The Doctor of Doctors
Lakshmi Gururajarao, M.D.

I offer my humble pranams at the lotus feet of Bhagavan Baba. I am blessed because, twenty-seven years ago, my husband introduced me to Swami. When I came to this country, I used to bow to Swami every day along with other deities in our prayer room. When I inquired about Baba, my husband gave me one of Mr. Howard Murphet's books to read, but I could not concentrate and, therefore, did not read it. My life changed within months after I had the opportunity to see a movie about Shirdi Sai Baba. I immediately understood that Baba was divine. I asked my husband to give me the book again and, this time, I read it. After reading about Sai Baba, I learned that Sai Baba and Shirdi Baba were one and the same. It was at that time that my husband told me about how a child's eyesight had been restored in Chicago. When the child had a penetrating eye injury, the mother of the child, who was our neighbor, asked him to pray. My husband gave her Swami's vibhuti to place on the child's forehead while uttering the name "Sai Ram" daily. Within a few days, the child recovered completely. This was a great surprise to me as well as to the doctors.

I have been a physician since 1969. I practiced in India three years before coming to the USA. In July, 1974, while being introduced to Swami's teachings, I began my residency training in Pediatrics. In December of that same year, my seventeen-month-old daughter came down with pneumonia. She was seen in the Emergency Room by doctors, put on antibiotics, and sent home. Within hours, she started to look worse, and when I took her back to the hospital, the repeat X-ray showed fluid in the pleural space (pleural effusion). She was then admitted into the hospital and started on intravenous antibiotics. She started to show intermittent nasal flaring and duskiness in the lips. On consultation with senior resident doctors who were on duty, I found out that they felt there was no need to aspirate the fluid; they thought antibiotics would be enough. However, I felt strongly that her lungs should be aspirated, otherwise she could go into respiratory distress. I felt helpless, started to cry, and told my husband about our daughter's condition. Immediately, he told me not to worry, and he sat in the conference room and started to pray. I remained with my daughter in the room.

Within fifteen to twenty minutes, a very dedicated senior pediatric surgeon walked into the room and asked me how everything was going. Immediately, I started crying and explained to the surgeon that the patient was my child. I told her all the details involving my daughter's condition. She requested that I show her the x-rays and, after reviewing them, she decided to tap the fluid from the lungs right away. She then informed the resident doctors about what she was going to do. After the procedure, my daughter's condition improved, her fever came down, and she started to play. She remained in the hospital for four weeks for intravenous antibiotics. My husband and I were very thankful to Swami.

When we were thanking the pediatric surgeon for her timely help, we found out that no one had called her to come into the hospital. It was a Sunday and, after attending church before returning home, she felt she wanted to stop at the hospital to check on things. She did not know why she came straight to the pediatric medical floor instead of, as usual, going directly to the pediatric surgical floor. When she saw me in the room, she entered and inquired if there were any problems. She was not aware that my daughter was a patient. It turned out my daughter had Staphylococcal Pneumonia, which is extremely rare and had not been seen for years in this institution. By Swami's grace, she recovered completely. After this, I continued to pray to Swami with more faith.

There was another incident that deepened and strengthened my faith in Swami. A family friend of mine had some guests from India, an elderly gentleman with his daughter. After visiting his son and on his way back to India, the gentleman wanted to visit my family friend. When she picked them up from the airport and took them home, she realized that they did not have their house key. They were unable to reach the supervisor of the building to ask for help. At the same time, they realized that the elderly gentleman had been sick during the flight. Therefore, my friend dropped her guests off at our home, explaining the situation to us, and went to search for the key. We welcomed her guests, and my husband immediately brought Swami's vibhuti from the prayer room and applied it on the gentleman's forehead as he uttered, "Sai Ram." Immediately, the daughter started to cry. We then found out that, for years, they had been staunch devotees of Swami. They were very happy to receive the vibhuti. When I went to examine the gentleman, I found out that he was having symptoms of a stroke. I immediately called our family physician who was kind enough to see him right away in his home office - on a Sunday! He was immediately admitted into the hospital for tests, as well as to control his blood sugar for diabetes and blood pressure for hypertension. Within a few days, he improved immensely and was picked up by his family. Thus, Swami took care of his devotee in a foreign country, in the best possible way, by not only giving comfort to his family during his illness, but by preventing him from having a major stroke.

In 1985, after thirteen years of knowing Swami, I had the opportunity to have His darshan in Whitefield in India. During the darshan, after Swami had not come to the ladies side at all for three days in a row, I prayed to Him, "Swami, how nice it would be if you could stand in the middle of the crowd, show your blessing hand, and bless everyone in all directions, so that everyone will be happy, as so many of us have traveled so far to come and have your darshan. Today you are passing the side where my husband is sitting. Please bless him, so the whole family will be blessed."

When we developed our film, in one of the exposures, Swami was passing my husband. In that picture, even though Swami was looking straight ahead, you could see that He was looking directly at my husband. In the photo, there was a ray of light passing from Swami's forehead into the sky, and a small standing image of Krishna was in that light. From this experience, I learned that Swami listens to everyone's prayers. Even though he does not appear to be looking at everyone, His vision goes out in all directions, and His blessings and divine energy flow to each and every person. From that time, I never worried about whether He came to the ladies side or not. A few times after that, He showered His grace on my family and me by giving us padnamaskar. Just knowing Swami is a great boon, and we do not need any other special blessing.

I have been practicing pediatrics for the last twenty-three years. In the beginning of my training, it used to upset me when I saw children with different last names in the same family, teenage pregnancy, children born out of wedlock, and drug addicted mothers. As I started to know Swami, and learn His teachings, my whole thought process changed. My views broadened, and I became more sensitive to the children and the needs of the families. I became more patient and able to listen to their needs and more tolerant and compassionate. I tried to be more accommodating, and, at the same time, educate them.

Before knowing Swami, when a patient came and complained that the medicine was not working or helping, I would get upset about the comment and take it personally. Now I listen carefully and look into the matter. I ask myself, why is the medicine not working for this child? I go into all the details and help the child and the parent by prescribing alternative medication, if necessary, or give other proper instructions. When children have chronic problems and physical disabilities, I now spend more time with the family and try to speak with love and empathy. In addition, I explore the possible ways to help the family and, many times, I bring prayer into my conversation by saying, "Let us pray together to win the Lord's grace." This often seems to satisfy the patient. I continue to pray to Swami, and I am grateful to Him for the transformation I am beginning to see in myself.

My practice is in an urban setting, so I often see mothers who are abusing alcohol and drugs. However, when the mothers are no longer abusing these substances, I am now able to see the love they have for their children by getting their children immunized and taking care of their health needs. Parents are sometimes very unreasonable about agreeing on treatments, or they are upset about their children's illness. By talking to them with love, I notice they calm down a lot.

I have a patient who was born with a chromosome abnormality. He has been admitted to the hospital many times. His mother did not speak English well, and his father got upset with everything and demanded a lot from the nursing staff and doctors. This was very difficult for everyone involved. By talking to the father, I realized that they were going through the stage of denial and, therefore, overreacting. So I tried to be more understanding and sympathetic and spent more time with them. I explained things in more detail, and I was available for them whenever they needed me. In due time, they started to change; they became more friendly, less demanding, and developed trust in what everyone was doing for them.

By acting in this manner, the patient/doctor relationship becomes smoother. I follow Swami's teachings to *Love All, Serve All,* and I try to see God in every human being. I also try not to judge any patient or family. I consider that all are God's children. It is difficult to describe but, in some instances, I see Swami's love in my patients. Swami's teachings have enabled me to work with more patience and tolerance. I find the nurses who work with me appreciate this.

When I am puzzled with a diagnosis of a patient's condition, I pray to Swami and ask for His guidance. Every morning I dedicate my thoughts, words, and actions to Swami before I start my work. I see that everything goes very smoothly in my practice, as well as in my daily life. Sometimes when medical problems arise, although they appear to be mountains, if I seek Swami's guidance, they melt like snow! Swami gives us clues. For example, I was treating a patient who was not doing well. All the work up we did on the patient did not help us arrive at a diagnosis. While I was thinking about this patient and getting worried, the words, "heart is enlarged" flashed into my mind. I did a chest X-ray and, to our surprise, the heart was enlarged. This led me to do more tests, thereby arriving at the proper diagnosis.

I feel Swami's omnipresence and see His hand in many instances. One of the premature infants has had multiple medical problems since birth, including major gastrointestinal problems. She was cared for by one of my colleague pediatricians, and a gastroenterologist was called in for consultation. During one of the multiple hospitalizations, my colleague was away, and I was covering. The day I started, the child's condition became worse. The kidney function tests were abnormal, and so the child was transferred to the Intensive Care Unit. When the physician in charge of the critical care unit explained about the possibility of permanent kidney damage, the parents were very upset. I started to pray to Swami for the child's recovery from kidney failure. Within a few days, the child recovered from the kidney failure completely. On transferring the patient back to the regular pediatric floor, the mother no longer wanted the child to be cared for by my colleague, so a different pediatrician took care of this child for the duration of the patient's stay in the hospital.

After a few months, my turn came for doing service rounds (taking care of in-patients who do not have a private pediatrician). My dilemma, at that time, was how should I take care of this patient? I knew that during my absence, the same colleague, whom the parents did not want, would have to take care of this child. A few days before I was about to start my service rounds, I prayed to Swami for guidance. On the day I was starting, I was standing near the nurses' station, and I was saying to myself, "Okay Swami, if it is Your will, I will take care of this patient, and You will take care of the rest." At that moment the telephone rang, and the gastroenterologist called out asking the resident physician to check if it was okay with me to transfer the patient to his service since the major problem was gastrointestinal. With tears in my eyes, I fervently thanked Swami and continued my rounds.

One thing in this world of which I am sure is the effectiveness of Swami's vibhuti. I have given it to sick people who have been given a poor prognosis and have seen a good outcome. Cancer patients have lived much longer then predicted, have less turbulent courses, and get mental and physical courage to face their illness. One patient with esophagus cancer and one with stomach cancer were given six months to live. They both had faith in God and took Swami's vibhuti. They both have lived more than eight years. I have also found that vibhuti has given comfort to the families. Every Thursday, when we have our family prayer, I pray for all the sick people, placing their names at His feet.

In my experience, prayer and vibhuti have been a very effective way of healing. Recently, I was asked to help plan the wedding of another Sai family member. The bride and groom, as well as their families, are also Sai devotees. On the morning of the wedding day, beginning at 4 a.m., the bride started to vomit every few seconds. Even though a physician, who was a relative, gave her medication, the vomiting did not stop. This made the family very anxious. When the make-up lady arrived to help her dress, she was not even able to sit. When I was leaving my house, after I went down a few steps, I was reminded to take some vibhuti with me. While I was on my way, the bride's parents were trying to reach me to ask for suggestions about their daughter's condition. When I arrived, I found the bride very weak, pale and dehydrated. Her head was bent down, and she was not paying attention to what was going on in the room. Immediately, I prayed to Swami, put the vibhuti in her mouth, held her hands and told her, "Let us pray together to Swami to stop this vomiting." Within five minutes, the whole picture changed. The color returned to her face, the nausea stopped, she started to sit up straight, and she even started to object to the color of the bangles the make-up lady was putting on her arms. She became very energetic. I had tears in my eyes as I thanked Swami. I told her mother to stay in the house, to get the bride ready, and not to worry any more. I proceeded to the wedding hall to take care of all the preparations. After two hours, the bride arrived for the wedding. She was radiant and full of energy. I learned later that she did not vomit at all after I left the house. Evidently, the make-up lady was very impressed and wanted to know to whom we had prayed. She wanted to know more about Swami. The wedding ceremony went beautifully. The bride reminded me of Mother Sita, Lord Rama's wife, full of beauty and radiance.

My thanks to Swami, the doctor of doctors, for his guidance, grace, and his never-ending help. I pray to Swami to bless me to continue to perform selfless service and to help me improve in my daily practice.

God is the embodiment of sweetness. Attain Him by offering Him who resides in all the sweetness that He has dowered on you. Crush the cane in the mill of Seva, boil it in the cauldron of penitence, decolorize of all sensual itch. Offer the crystallized sugar of compassionate love to Him.

Sathya Sai Baba, *Sathya Sai Speaks, Volume II*

Transformation

S. K. Upadhyay, M.B.B.S., D.O.M.S., M.R.C. Ophth.

I have been practicing medicine for 32 years. I qualified as a doctor in 1968. Since 1974, I have specialized in Ophthalmology. I love restoring sight. After surgery, when the bandages come off, and the patient's open their eyes and can see nature—a gift of God they had been deprived of—they totally believe that God exists.

In 1974, I had the wonderful opportunity to come to the UK to do my studies and continue my practice. My work is divided into three areas: I work for the National Health Service, a government hospital; I have a private practice in Harley Street; and I devote a large amount of time traveling abroad to developing countries. I arrange eye camps in many parts of the world including Africa, Russia, India, Sri Lanka, Bangladesh and many other areas where there is need. We have a wonderful team of volunteers. They go out with me and experience that service to man is service to God.

It was in 1970 when I came face to face with the reality of Sathya Sai Baba for the first time. I was working in the Himalayas with a colleague who was a radiologist. It was extremely cold, and in the winter months the temperature fell to well below zero. We lived in bunkers in very ordinary conditions. In order to prevent the loss of heat, these bunkers are lined with parachute material, and to keep the bunker warm, we burned kerosene in drums. On a shelf, my friend had a picture of Sai Baba and some deities. I also worshipped Rama, Krishna and Shiva and, after my bath, offered my prayers and chanted the Gayatri mantra. But, somehow, I could not believe that Sai Baba was divine and God incarnate. My friend told me it didn't matter who I believed in. He said that as long as I followed the right path, Sai Baba would be happy with me. He gave me vibhuti daily, which I took reluctantly. I took it because I'd been taught to respect all faiths and religions, because they imbibed the principle of love all, serve all. One day, when we returned to our bunker, we found that there had been a fire and everything had been burned. We had some metal trunks where we kept our valuables. Even those were completely melted and nothing was left. I was very surprised to see that only Sai Baba's picture and a

couple of other pictures, as well as my Ophthalmology book
where I had kept a picture of Baba that my friend had given me,
were still intact. As a doctor and a scientist, I thought there must
be something very significant about a fire where each and every
thing, including a metal trunk, was destroyed and where only
these few items remained. This event brought about a slight
change of heart about Baba, but I was still not 100% convinced.

A year passed, and I was posted in central India. As a part of
our training, we had to go into the villages and help in the medical
camps. I did not realize that working in these camps and helping
the poor would become the ultimate reality of my life. It was
during this period that I had two serious accidents which could
have left me paralyzed or with head injuries. Although my
motorbike was destroyed, I received no permanent injuries. It was
then that I realized I was under a divine umbrella and God was
protecting me.

It was in 1982 that I came face to face with the Lord. The first
time I went to Prasanthi Nilayam I did not get an interview, but
Swami gave a discourse in the afternoon that changed my life. I
had so many questions and thought if I had a chance to speak to
Sai Baba, I would ask him these questions. To my utter surprise,
He opened His discourse with a beautiful Telegu poem and, then,
said that there were many people present who had doubts about
His divinity. He told us that we are all the embodiment of the
same divine power; that is why He calls us embodiments of
divine love. The problem was that we were all looking for God
outside. He said that we waste our time searching for God by
going to the mountains and the caves and seeking information
from sages and saints,. He said that He has realized He is God but
that we still doubt our divinity. I was shocked because this was
exactly what I felt. One of the reasons I wanted to be posted in the
high altitude regions was that I wanted to meet some sages and
people who had been doing penance in the Himalayas. I wanted to
sit down and ask them how I could realize divinity. I had also
wondered how Sai Baba, who is like any other human being
walking on this planet, could be God? Here was Sai Baba

answering my questions. It was an eye opener for me. Since then, I have never looked back.

Sai Baba's influence has played a great role in my practice. I can recollect very clearly that we had an opportunity to conduct a medical camp during Swami's sixtieth birthday in 1986 in the villages around Puttaparthi. Doctors from countries all over the world came to offer their services for this occasion. I was very lucky to be selected, and our team was the only one that was given the chance to do surgery. The village that was chosen was Bukkapatnum, very close to Puttaparthi and the place where Swami had His primary school education. This school had been converted into a clinic. Every morning, the doctors and volunteers would meet in the Hill View Stadium. Swami would come, break a coconut and sprinkle the water over us. Then, we would all go to work in the villages.

At the end of the camp, we were very lucky because Swami granted all of us a 90 minute interview. He gave us the beautiful insight of what a doctor should be like. He said that love and compassion are the two most important ingredients that patients look for in a doctor. He told us we may be wonderful surgeons or doctors, but if we do not have love and compassion, a patient will not be very happy to see us. He said that we first have to win the confidence of the patient. We are not to worry about what we gain from the patient. We must offer our services without any reward. He told us that most doctors have the problem of thinking about what are they going to get in monetary terms, and their behavior changes if the patient cannot afford to pay. *They offer a very quick service,* Swami said. *Do not go for this two-tier system.*

I remember, before I came to Sai Baba, I used to attend many medical camps and was very much duty bound. I would finish my work and come home. I thought I had finished my duty and was happy I had given my services to the poor. I did not have a personal relationship with the patients on whom I operated. Also, I did not care about the surroundings we worked in or where the patients were kept or where we operated on them. In those days, because of cost-effectiveness, the camps were arranged in schools and tents.

Swami gave me an insight by saying, *What you cannot offer to your mother and father, brother and sister, do not offer to a poor person.* He told us to have the same standard for the poor and the rich and not to offer inferior treatment like outdated medicine or treatment in a tent. We are to maintain a high quality of surgery for all, as we do in England, because God lives in everyone. This was really a wonderful teaching for me and has changed my entire viewpoint. Ever since then, I have changed my style of work. We still go to the villagers in remote parts of the world, but now we use the best possible equipment for diagnosis. We no longer perform surgery in tents and under poor conditions as we did before. The patients are now brought by car or coaches to the nearest hospital or nursing home and are given proper after care as well.

Another thing Swami introduced into our consciousness is that it is very important to follow up these cases. I never thought about what happened to these patients after their operations. I presumed they were well looked after. As we do in England, we give the best surgery with the most advanced technology and, now, there are always doctors left behind to see if there are any complications. I am very pleased to say that whenever we have done any of the camps with the Sai Organization, I have not seen any complications. Sometimes Baba sends His divine help to us and, later on, when we get to see Him, He will jokingly ask, *Did you receive my help?* It has given us strength knowing that He is constantly working with us and watching over us.

Although Swami may not have been physically present, I have known many incidents that go on in the camps which He later explained, in detail, in an interview. Once, a medical camp was arranged near the famous village of Shirdi. During the camp, a very old, poor, and sick lady was examined by one of the team doctors. He asked her to get a chest X-ray to confirm his diagnosis. A few days later, when we arrived at Ooti, Swami very kindly granted us an interview. He explained how an ideal medical camp is arranged, how medicines should be distributed, and how doctors should conduct themselves, giving their skills and their love. He spoke like a professor of science. He then narrated the incident just described, in detail, saying that the poor lady should not have been sent for an X-ray, because it was a clear case of Tuberculosis. She had all the signs and symptoms of the disease including her appearance, emaciated body, cough and fever. He said that if she had the money for an x-ray, she would have used it to treat the disease with medicines in the first place. He then explained what method of treatment should have been undertaken. He may be sitting hundreds of miles away but, in spirit, He is still watching and guiding us. This has greatly enhanced my faith in His omnipresence.

Before Swami came into my life, I used to go to the hospital and, when I was about to finish my duty, if another patient came in, I would try to turn him over to the next colleague on duty. Now, it no longer matters what time I finish at the hospital. I am just happy and feel privileged that I have been given the opportunity to see another person.

My attitude toward patients has also changed. I have become extremely friendly with them. I no longer bother about time. Because of my attitude, many patients, particularly the elderly ones, have become like family members. They have faith in me and discuss all their problems, not only about their eyes. This is something I treasure.

I used to have difficulties with my nursing staff and some colleagues. This was perhaps due to my Army training; I would lose my temper quickly if I didn't see things done the way I wanted. This had caused a problem with the staff. After that interview with Swami, I came home thinking that all the people working with me are also divine. The surroundings completely changed. The change was so profound that I could feel His grace working. One nurse, who didn't get along with anyone, changed her attitude and became a friend. Now, she provides me with everything I need. Since I came into close physical contact with Swami and touched His lotus feet, I feel a great deal of love and compassion within me. Service has become devotion to me. I am serving the Lord through my patients.

On one occasion, one of my colleagues at the clinic was supposed to examine a blind gentleman who was also on insulin.

Everyone thought there was nothing much that could be done for him. My colleague was overstressed and got very angry and started shouting when he learned that the man had forgotten to bring his urine sample. This poor man became very frightened and left the clinic. When he went to the Institute for the Blind, he was given my name and told he must have his eyes checked. However, he was scared to go back to the clinic. I came to know of this and approached him saying, "Please brother, don't go to the same clinic; come to me and we will examine your eyes."

Notice how Swami sets the drama. Because I did not know anything about this man, I started the examination from scratch. Recently, there had been a lot of developments in technology and procedures had improved. I realized that something could be done for this man. I felt that there was a chance he might be able to see. He experienced the intense love in my practice, and I remember him saying, "It doesn't matter if I can see or not, but I am so happy there is someone who can talk to me so lovingly. My wife left me; I have no children; I live alone and hardly anyone visits; I've lost all my friends." Despite his extreme shortsightedness and the diabetes, there was great potential for him, so we performed the surgery. I am very happy to say that, even though he is an old man, he can now see and read very well. He cried while expressing his gratitude. I told him, "Don't thank me, thank Sai Baba." When he learned about Swami, he started attending bhajans. He can go by bus and he now has many Sai friends. People visit him, take him for outings, and he attends bhajans regularly. This has totally changed his life. This is how the principle of love can bring not only reward to the patient but a great deal of satisfaction to the surgeon.

Since I have come into the Sai fold, the moment I enter the operating theater (OT) or am about to see a patient, I always pray: "Make me an instrument and help me cure or help this patient." When I used to enter the OT, there was tension before the operation or during the procedure if there was a complication. This would show in my behavior and I would become a little irritable. But ever since coming to Swami, I have found a great deal of calmness. I offer my prayers and surrender totally to the

Lord. When I handle the knife, I no longer feel any tension. I used to get nervous but with prayer, or keeping Sai Baba's locket on my neck, or having a picture of Sai in front of me, I feel very relaxed.

However, in the past there were many occasions where I was in doubt about what decision to make. He has made it very simple for me. I close my eyes and say, "Swami, what should I do?" The reply comes, "Would you do it for your mother or father. If yes, then go ahead and do it." I never have had any problems since then. Swami's ultimate teaching is, *Service to man is service to God.* When you are serving your fellow man, you no longer think that you are serving the person who is sitting in front of you. You think that your service to your patient is reaching Swami. This fundamental teaching has changed my attitude toward the patient. I no longer have to worry about making a decision, because I know, if these principles are in front of me, I will always make the right decision.

There was one incident after an operation where a gentleman had lost his eyesight in one eye and started losing sight in his other eye afterward. Somehow, he found out about the compassionate work that we render for free. He started ringing me. I was out of the country, and he probably thought I was avoiding him. One day he phoned and, threatening, told my wife that if I don't see him, he would commit suicide. When I finally saw him, I realized he was a desperate young man. He clearly told me that if his eyesight was not restored, he had nothing left to live for. All his friends had left him, and he was living in extreme poverty. I was worried and started praying. I did not know what to do. I felt I had no choice but to perform the surgery, otherwise he would commit suicide. I explained that we would do an operation but that he should not hope for a miracle immediately. It might take a very long time. I told him he must remove from his mind the idea of killing himself. Meanwhile, I was intensely and desperately praying: "Swami, You have put me in this situation. Please help me so that this man does not kill himself." We performed the operation on his eye and asked him to come in a week later. To my utter surprise, his eyesight was immediately and completely restored.

At this point, I realized it was not my surgery or the medical intervention. It must have been his karma and the direct intervention of Swami. He definitely listened to my prayer. After seeing this result, the patient forced us to do an operation on his other eye, which was already damaged. Eventually, the vision also improved in that eye, although not to the same extent as the first eye. Now, with the grace of God, he has normal vision in both eyes. He is working and driving. One day when this man was present, I was explaining to friends about the grace of God. My friends challenged me by asking if I trusted him to drive me. I told them that I had total faith and gave him my car keys. We drove to a Sai meeting in Leicester about 100 miles from London. He confidently drove me there. I had no fear whatsoever. My main idea was to take him to a Sai meeting and introduce him to Sai. Later on, he told me that in childhood he had had an incident when he was drowning and that Shirdi Sai Baba had saved his life.

There are many incidents in my practice here and abroad where I have had a direct intervention by the divine power. There was a boy, whom I met with a colleague, who was diagnosed with leukemia and only given about a year to live. They started chemotherapy. He lost his eyebrows and hair, was vomiting, and had other complications. The family was told he did not have a good prognosis. The parents thought that if the chemotherapy was not going to work and the child only had a short time to live, what was the point of torturing him. This family was told about Sai Baba and given some vibhuti. Their faith worked, and the child recovered. He had a total remission. Now, he is grown up and working happily.

I have noticed that many people have been influenced by Swami's teachings, not just by His miracles. When I give talks on health, education, social reform, and Swami sending advanced technologies into remote parts of the world, many doctors show interest in joining me in the medical camps. I remember that one of the well-known doctors practicing in Wimpole Street decided to come with me to one of the medical camps. When he saw the volunteers and doctors doing selfless service to humanity, starting their work at 4:00 am and working sometimes to 2:00 am in the morning, he knew something special was happening. When he saw them doing all their work with a smile and not complaining about the lack of food or sleep, he realized there was an extraordinary force working behind all these people. At the end, when he saw the joy and love that brought people together, he realized Sai must be this divine force. He then decided to go and see Swami.

For the past 22 years, I have worked with an eye specialist who had been my consultant and teacher. He is a top ophthalmology scholar—the best in his field. As my teacher, he taught me a wonderful eye surgery technique. With Swami's grace, I have taken this technology to several poverty stricken areas.

I had a deep desire for my old teacher to meet Sai Baba some day. But, he had a rather grand notion of Sai Baba's ashram. He imagined it was like the Vatican. He thought that when he got there, he would have an interview and sit down and talk with Swami. My teacher has operated on the eyes of many very important people in the world. Wherever he goes, he is greeted with great respect and receives red-carpet treatment. He expected the same to happen when he met Sai Baba. I tried to explain that it wouldn't happen that way. Sai Baba's way was very different.

Thanks to an organization called Care and Share International Research Foundation, we acquired a new machine that gives instant relief to cataract sufferers. It is especially beneficial for poor people, since a person can have a cataract operation in the morning and go back to work the same day. Thus, a breadwinner doesn't lose wages and deprive his family of much-needed income. A training program to learn how to use this machine was arranged at the Super Specialty Hospital.

On my next trip to Prasanthi Nilayam, Swami finally agreed that the professor should accompany me. When I broke the news to my teacher, he was very excited. He then instructed me to book him into the best five star hotel—with a swimming pool.

Alarmed, I tried to explain, "Sir, we are going to visit a beautiful, divine ashram. We won't be in a five-star hotel. The only swimming pool will be the pool of love."

"Oh, I'm sure there's a big town nearby," he replied. I mentioned Bangalore. "How far is it?" he asked.

"A hundred miles."

"Fine. I drive that far every day from my home in Camberly to London. I can stay in Bangalore and drive to the hospital in Puttaparthi every morning."

I tried to describe driving in India, which is **not** the equivalent of a trip from his home to London. But my teacher wasn't sure he wanted to stay in the ashram. I was worried. As the time approached, my excitement at taking him to see Swami turned to nervousness. I prayed. "Swami, I am bringing my teacher, but I don't know if he will fit into your discipline. Should we cancel the trip?"

Our plans were to leave on November 4th, but when I called the professor on November 1st, I found out that he was in Gibraltar. He returned November 3rd and I asked if he had his visa. "No, you are arranging the visa."

"How can I arrange a visa without your passport?" Secretly, I was relieved because now I thought I could cancel the trip. Then I remembered someone who could obtain a special visa for him. But the professor dropped a bombshell: his wife wanted to come too. I figured I could arrange for one person to stay in a nice place in Puttaparthi, but men and women together are always a problem there, and his wife had never even been to a Sai meeting. I was worried. I said, "Where is her passport?"

"It's in Camberly," he replied. "She will fax you the information."

"Sorry," I told him. "The High Commission won't issue a visa on a faxed passport." "But I **must** go. Swami is calling me," he replied.

"Then Swami will have to perform a miracle," I said.

Immediately, two things happened. One of our dear friends came to see me, and I asked them to pray for me because I was so nervous. Fifteen minutes later, the High Commissioner of India came to see us. He told me that he heard that I was leaving town, and he wanted to consult about his eye problem before we left. I assured him that we would only be gone for a few days, but he insisted that something had told him to come today.

"I will have to see you later on," I said. "I have a problem."

"What's the problem?" he asked.

I explained that I urgently needed visas. He made one phone call and forty minutes later we had visas. That's how Swami works. But I still had some worries because I had overheard the professor ask his wife to go to an expensive London shop to buy wine to take to India. "Is that necessary?" I asked him.

"You said there were no good drinks available there, so we want to take our own," he said.

"But you can't drink in the ashram."

"Why not? When I was with the Bishop, he shared wine with me," he replied.

"But you are going to the divine," I said. "'De' and 'vine' means no wine!"

He told me not to worry, that everything would be all right. I was worried and praying.

When I got home that night, my wife showed me a fax that had come through our friend, Lucas Ralli. It was a beautiful message, "My son, why worry? He is my guest. I will look after him." I felt as if a burden had been lifted. I sat right down and thanked Swami. But He continued to test me. Within an hour, the professor called to ask if we were going first class. I told him our group always travels economy to save money. "You should have told me," he said. "I never travel economy class. I'll take my checkbook to the airport and change my seat." I told him I doubted that he could make a last minute change. He sounded very unhappy. To make matters worse, at the airport the next morning, all our hospital paraphernalia put us far over the weight allowance—by 200 pounds!

"We **must** take everything," I told the Air India receptionist. "It is all for Swami. If you don't send it, we can't perform eye operations."

The receptionist said she would see what she could do. Soon after, she asked, "Are Dr. and Mrs. A. in your group?"

"Yes."

"Fine," she said. "They are first class passengers and are allowed the additional weight."

"How did they get first class tickets?" I asked.

"I don't know," she replied. "I just received a fax saying they had been promoted to first class." Everything was in order. Swami had arranged for the professor's upgrade.

After a long trip, we reached Puttaparthi at 4:15 p.m. Everyone in the Accommodations and Public Relations Office was in the mandir for Swami's darshan. We left the taxi outside and went inside the mandap. One of our doctor friends, who lives mostly in Prasanthi, was coordinating our trip. He was very worried about what to do next, because everyone he knew was sitting on the veranda. But a volunteer helped us and took us right in, as Swami was amongst the devotees giving darshan and collecting letters. We were guided near Swami's room where we sat down. The professor was sweating and puffing in his best suit and tie. Everyone was looking at him, wondering who was this man in a Western suit. The professor was also concerned about his wife's whereabouts.

Swami came out and asked us to come inside where some friends of ours from Russia were also waiting. Swami asked the professor how he was.

"Sir, I am fine," he replied. He spoke to Swami as if He were a person, calling Him "sir."

Swami said that since the professor wasn't used to sitting cross-legged, he could stretch his legs out. *There are no restrictions here*, He said, *So you can be comfortable. Inside here you are all right.* Swami was very kind. He switched on the fan, and we sat down.

I wanted to speak to Swami about the professor's accommodation problem. I began, "Swami, he..."

Swami interrupted me, *You keep quiet. Do not talk.* So I kept quiet. Then, Swami turned His attention to a young Russian who was sitting next to Swami's chair. He materialized a beautiful ring upon which was carved the sacred Om. Instead of giving the ring to the young man, Swami tossed it to the professor who caught it. *What do you think it is?* Swami asked.

He looked at the ring and said, "I don't know exactly what it is, sir, but it is some sort of holy sign. I recognize it because Dr. Upadhyay uses it each time he starts something new."

Swami said, *In the West, you say that the world started with a big bang. This is the same primordial sound that the whole world came from. It is called Om. Say it with Me. Om.*

I did not realize that Swami was doing this to initiate him. At that moment, the professor was sitting with his legs stretched toward Swami. I was very uncomfortable because I didn't think that was right. But the moment I tried to open my mouth, Swami silenced me, *Keep quiet.* Suddenly, as the professor said "Om," his stretched legs folded, his hands came together in reverence and he said, "Yes, Swami." The transformation was total. Swami took the ring from the professor and started to give it to the Russian boy, knowing full well that the boy did not want a ring with Om.

What do you want? Swami asked.

The Russian boy replied, "Swami, I want Your picture on the ring." Swami took the ring and, one foot away from the professor's face, blew on it changing it into a beautiful ring with His picture on it. He put the ring on the boy's middle finger, and then He started talking to the group. After a while, he told us that we should start the operations and train Super Specialty Hospital doctors in the new technique. Gradually, everyone got up and began to go out.

"Where is the professor going to stay?" I asked Swami.

He smiled, *There is no problem. He will stay in the ashram.* I also asked about the wine and He said, *Leave it outside.* I didn't understand what He meant. He added, *Come tomorrow morning; I will give more instructions.*

It was the first time I had left Swami's room utterly confused. Here He was telling me to stay in the ashram, yet the professor had said he didn't want to stay there. I thought I had to arrange a place with air-conditioning at least—even if it wasn't a five-star hotel. But when I went to join the professor, he said, "It's foolish of me to think about staying somewhere else. I will stay in the ashram. I just want a room with a toilet, a bathroom and a fan. That's all, nothing else." Total transformation! Before the interview, he **had** to have a room with air-conditioning. After 15 minutes with Swami, everything had changed.

"What about your wine?" I asked.

"Let the taxi man have it," he said. "Just get our luggage and leave everything else outside." That was what Swami had meant by, *Leave it outside.* The taxi driver got the gift of a lifetime.

The next morning, when we came for darshan, Swami had made wonderful arrangements for us to sit near His door.

The professor asked, "Is it possible for my wife to see Swami also?"

"That's up to Swami," I answered. "We don't even know yet if He will see you."

"But Swami said He would see me," the professor replied.

"When Swami says He'll see you tomorrow, His tomorrows are sometimes very long," I told him. "It could be next year; it could be next life. He may see you. He may not see you."

"No," he said. "This morning I prayed deep inside, and I could hear Swami say, 'Yes. Both of you.'"

"Let's see what happens," I said.

Then Swami came and asked both of us to go inside. The professor whispered, "Ask about my wife."

"You don't have to ask God for anything. He knows everything." But Swami did not give us a chance to speak further.

Suddenly, He turned to us, *Yes, yes, call your wife*, He said. Since his wife had never been to the interview room, she didn't know what to do. She sat down between her husband and me. Swami leaped from His chair and said, *Wife, this is an ashram, not London. You do not sit with men.* She went to the women's side and sat down.

Swami talked to several people, then he turned to the professor's wife. *What do you want?* He asked.

I couldn't imagine why Swami would ask her this question, because she had never known about Sathya Sai Baba. I had no idea what she would say. To my utter surprise, she responded, "Swami, I do not want anything. After looking at you, I just want Your grace."

Swami materialized a beautiful pendant with His picture on it and gave it to her. Then He turned to the professor and materialized a ring for him saying, *This ring is a communication ring. Whenever you want to speak to me, speak through it.* As the professor stared at the ring, I nudged him to pay attention. Swami continued, *It took so long for you to come to me. You have been thinking of coming for the last 25 years. The time has come. You are a kind man. Now work for mankind.*

How Swami plays with words! Then Swami took them both to the inner room. After 20 minutes, they came out and He said, *Go straight to the operation theater.* I asked the professor to wait for me since Swami had told me to stay back.

What is your problem now? Swami asked me.

"No problem Swami. I leave everything to you." Then He spoke at length about the eye operations and the new machines. *Make sure that every evening I get a report of what is happening,* He said. *Also, make sure that before you leave, my surgeons are as well trained as you two so that they can do this operation on their own.* I was about to tell Swami that it took us years to learn the skills; I was going to ask Him how His doctors could possibly learn it in three days. But before I could speak, Swami said, *Do not worry about time and space.*

When we came out, we passed a woman sitting in a wheelchair. Swami asked her why she had not come inside.

"Swami, You closed the door," she said, "And no one was here to lift me up in my wheelchair."

Wheelchair? Why are you in a wheelchair? He asked.

"Swami, I can't walk," she said.

Who said you cannot walk? Swami was standing outside the interview room with 10,000 people watching. He extended His lovely hand to the woman and said, *Hold my hand and get up.* The woman stood up and Swami pushed the wheelchair away. *You can walk now.*

The professor was absolutely astonished by all he had seen. He didn't know what to say. He did manage to say simply, "Swami, it would be nice if you could come to the operating theater."

Oh, yes, I will be there.

We went directly to the Super Specialty Hospital, changed, scrubbed, and went to the operating theater where a patient and all the instruments were ready. But the professor sat, waiting.

"What are you waiting for?" I asked.

"Where is Swami? he asked, "He said He was coming."

"Yes," I said. "Swami said He was coming. He **is** here, but not necessarily in physical form."

"No, no. He told me He was coming." And the professor— with six patients waiting and a staff eager to finish work so they could go to afternoon darshan—refused to start.

So I said to him, "Okay, you start and I will find out what's happening." So I changed again and went outside. Several doctors and some Care and Share people from London were waiting in the lounge to see the operation performed live on the monitor. I needed to speak to Swami. But you can't just pick up the phone and call Him. I went into the little shrine room outside the Operating Theater and prayed, "Swami, he is not starting without You. Please do something. Either come Yourself or just give him the vision to start the operation." Then I headed back to the operating room.

When I walked in, the professor turned to me, "I think we should start. Swami will probably come halfway through. He is very busy." I thanked Swami.

During the operation, something unusual happened. After the cataract is crushed and washed, the next step is to insert a new lens called an implant. A nurse in the room had in her case fifteen British-made implants. She opened a fresh pack and rinsed one in distilled water to make sure it was clean. Then we put it under a microscope to look at it. The moment the professor lifted the implant, Baba was there. For the first time, I could see tears in his eyes. Again, total transformation. For a moment, he was speechless. Then he told me he would finish the operation, but I would have to instruct the doctors on the procedure. "I simply cannot speak," he said. "I am in total bliss." This comment was recorded on the video that was being made as a training tool. He finished the operation beautifully and found that Swami had left him a message, *Do not rush back; carry on the second session also. I will see you tomorrow.* We proceeded with all the operations. Swami had selected very poor people – those who could never even dream of having expensive eye surgery.

If you saw the professor at work as a private surgeon in England, you would see a madhouse. Patients and doctors from every nation in the world come to confer with him. Normally, a person waits hours to see him. Yet here he was, operating on the world's poorest people with great happiness and bliss. He was a totally transformed man. After the session, he told me something very beautiful. "I have operated on some of the richest men in the world," he said, "But I did not get this much satisfaction. Today, after operating on people so poor that they don't even have decent clothes to wear, I feel I offered something to God."

Afterward, Swami spoke to him and said He would see him again. The 24-hour Akhanda Bhajan had just started in the mandir. The professor came and sat with me. As before, he had put on his new suit. I asked him why he didn't wear something more comfortable—a simple kurta pajama or light trousers.

"No," he replied. "I heard Sai Baba tell someone, *'Do not try to change yourself. Be yourself.'* Do I ever wear kurta pajamas in England? No. If I go to meet the queen or the Pope or the President of the United States, I go in the best suit possible. I am going to meet the Lord. It doesn't matter whether I feel comfortable or uncomfortable. I should be in my best suit."

The bhajans started, and the professor sat waiting for Swami. After an hour and a half, I noticed that his legs were getting cramped from sitting cross-legged for so long. I said, "I'm sure Swami won't speak to you until tomorrow when the bhajans are over. Why don't you go ahead on your trip." He and his wife were scheduled to go to Bangalore so she could do some shopping. Afterward, they planned to go to Ooty and Mysore to see some historic places. Since the professor had performed an operation on one of the members of a wealthy family in Mysore, he had been invited to visit. While he was away, I planned to stay and enjoy the bhajans.

At eight o'clock, realizing that Swami would not see him that night, the professor left for Bangalore with his wife. But the next morning, he said to his wife, "I don't feel like going out. I have come here for a purpose – not for sightseeing or shopping or visiting a family. You go ahead; I would like to sit here and read some Baba books." His wife left with a friend, and the professor stayed in the hotel reading a Baba book. That evening, they went to bed early. But at ten, the professor awoke suddenly and asked his wife if she had heard anything.

"Yes," she said. "I heard Baba say, 'Come back.'" He had heard the same thing, "Come back," said very clearly from a corner of the room. They agreed that the next morning, instead of going to Ooty, they would return to Puttaparthi.

Meanwhile, when the bhajans finished, Swami gave us beautiful prasad with His own hands. Suddenly, He said to me, *Start the operation at eight a.m. tomorrow. He is coming back.* I was surprised because this was not the schedule in our program, but I was sure this was Swami's will.

The professor and his wife got up at four in the morning and arrived back at the ashram at 7:59. Swami told us to go to the hospital right after darshan. *Everything is waiting for you,* He said. When we got there, we understood the reason we were needed: the surgeons still were not confident enough to do the operation on their own. We worked very hard all day. At about four in the afternoon, we asked the head doctor if he felt more confident now.

"Yes, now I am happy," he replied. We asked him to do an operation on his own, and we watched while he performed it perfectly. We rushed to Swami. Like a mother, he was waiting. Darshan was over, but we got there in time to take pad-namaskar.

Then Swami explained, *I called you because I knew they were not ready to do the operation independently. Now the program is complete. That is why I said to him, 'I'll see you.'* The professor had been worried Swami would not see him before we left for home. He took Swami's padnamaskar. Then Swami said, *Do not worry. This is your home. You can come anytime.* And He blessed us.

The professor is now working to organize a mission that will take Swami's message and the new technology from village to village. I have seen a transformation. The professor—a material man—has become so humble that he wants to devote his time to mankind. When Swami touches someone, the transformation can be complete.

These experiences and Swami's teachings have totally transformed my life and changed my attitude in my practice. I feel very fortunate that Swami entered into my life and totally transformed me and made me His instrument to serve the community the way He wants me to serve. I pray that He continues to shower His grace to allow me to work for Him.

The story of the professor was based on a talk given by Dr. Upadhyay at an Interfaith Meeting in London on June 20, 1998, and previously published in the June issue of *Sai Sarathi*.

Doctors have to endeavor to become the receptacles of divine power during their healing process. How can they heal when they themselves are ill, either in body or mind? When their minds are innocent and contented, a smile will spontaneously shine on their faces, and their words will be soft, sweet and tender, softer than any pharmaceutical balm. The manner and mien of the physician are more effective in drawing out the latent sources of strength in the patient than the most powerful drug. A prayerful atmosphere of humility and veneration will go a long way to help the cure. We may say that the behavior, the voice, the mien of the doctor count for fifty percent of the cure; the drugs and their efficacy manage the other half.

Sathya Sai Baba
Sanathana Sarathi, Vol. 23 #9, September 1980, pp 200-201

Putting Sai Baba's Teachings into Practice
Joseph G. Phaneuf, M.D.

I began my studies at Macomb Community College in Michigan after returning from active duty in the Naval Air Force Reserves in 1970. I had been trained as an airplane mechanic and continued to work at Selfridge Naval Air Force Base as an airplane mechanic one weekend a month for the next five years. After one year at *Macomb*, I transferred to Western Michigan University and began a premed program. School was hard work, but I did very well. I was proud of the fact that I got straight A's. At this stage in life, I definitely thought that I was the doer and felt that hard work was all that was necessary to be successful in life. I had a hard time understanding why my friends were having a difficult time just getting passing grades when I was doing so well. I didn't realize that God had blessed me with the ability to do well in school. I felt that if my friends just studied harder, they could also get good grades like me. I believed that the end result of my education was to get into a good medical school. I thought that the overall purpose of education was to get an interesting and good paying job. However, I have learned over the years that education has a much higher purpose. As Sai Baba has told us, *The end of education is character.*

I began medical school in 1974 at the University of Michigan. I first heard about Sai Baba around 1975 from a friend who lived in a basement apartment just down the hall from me. She gave me a book called *Sai Baba, The Holy Man and the Psychiatrist* by Dr. Samuel Sandweiss. I looked at the picture on the front cover and thought Sai Baba's picture was actually a picture of the author and figured this psychiatrist, in the orange robe with the big Afro hairdo, was a bit weird. Unfortunately, I didn't read this book until several years later.

I finished medical school in 1978, did a one-year medical internship, then three years of dermatology training. In July 1982, I started to work in private practice as a dermatologist in a small town in Texas. In 1993, I moved to Northern California and began to work as a dermatologist for Kaiser Permanente, a large, non-profit HMO, one of the few awarded for its excellence in managed care.

Soon after starting college, I attended a lecture on the Transcendental Meditation technique founded by Mahareshi Mahesh Yogi. I noticed good results and continued to practice this meditation technique for the next twelve years. This technique was a great diffuser of stress for me. Ever since I started to practice TM, I was intent on finding the most enlightened person on earth who could help me on my spiritual path. At first, I thought that Mahareshi Mahesh Yogi was the one. But over the years, I learned he was not the one I was seeking. I finally found the person I was looking for in a most interesting way. In 1985, I was talking with a friend in my kitchen. I was still doing Transcendental Meditation and was talking about how powerful the TM siddhis program was. This was an advanced TM technique to develop super normal powers. I explained that if 7000 people were practicing the TM siddhis program all in one place, it could bring about profound changes such as peace in a war zone like the Middle East. Much to my surprise, my friend stated, "I know someone who can do that very easily just by willing it." I asked her who that could be, and she said, "Sai Baba."

We talked some more about Sai Baba, and I began to read about Him. I soon realized that Sai Baba was the one that I had been looking for all along. I was also beginning to become disenchanted with the TM technique. First of all, there was a fee to be able to learn the technique, which was not cheap and, therefore, not everyone who wanted to learn could afford it. Sai Baba voiced what my conscience had been telling me, that there should be no charge for spiritual instruction. Also, much of what I learned from TM residence courses was supposed to be kept secret, and this bothered me a lot. I did not think that spiritual information should be kept secret. Sai Baba also validated this feeling when I read about him saying that spiritual information should be available to everyone, and no information of this type should be kept secret. To add to this, my experience with meditation was getting very time consuming. I was spending about two hours each day in meditation, and I felt that my time could be spent in better ways. I also felt that, even though I had become good at dealing with stress, my heart was dry. Sai Baba says we should meditate on God all day long, and that being of service to others is more important than sitting for hours crossed legged and repeating a mantra. So I stopped practicing TM. This gave me a new focus for my life. I realized that being a good person and serving others at work and at home was more important than praying or meditating. As Sai Baba says, *Hands that serve are holier than lips that pray.* However, Swami still advocates prayer and meditation but emphasizes that service to others should be our main focus. Recently, I started to practice the light meditation as recommended by Sai Baba. This only takes a small amount of time each morning and night. Learning this meditation is free of charge and is easy for almost anyone to learn.

In 1986, I visited Sai Baba for the first time. At one of the first darshans, Swami came up to me, asked where I was from, and materialized vibhuti for me. This was the start of my spiritual awakening.

I went to visit the Sathya Sai General Hospital, which is adjacent to the ashram, and volunteered to work there. This hospital gives medical care to anyone who needs it, and the doctors who work there do so free of charge. The doctors are given free room and board but no salary. The doctors are top notch, compassionate, and hard working. When I showed up at the hospital to volunteer, the medical director asked me what I wanted. I explained that I was a dermatologist from the USA, and I would like to see patients that had skin problems. The first thing I was asked to do was to read a x-ray. Since I am a dermatologist, I thought this was a bit strange; but luckily, I read the x-ray satisfactorily and was allowed to see one patient who was a student at Swami's school in Puttaparthi. I did not see any other patients during this trip.

Subduing the Ego

It was at this point that Baba began to slowly work on subduing my ego. Actually, I did not think that I had a big ego. I know doctors are known for having big egos but, compared to them, I thought I was very humble. Right away, a Sai Baba devotee told me that I was perhaps the only Western doctor that had been allowed to work in the Sathya Sai General Hospital except for Dr. Sam Sandweiss. "Wow, that's great," I thought. I felt very special and was happy that I was recognized in this way.

My next visit to see Swami was two years later in 1988. One night, while staying in a shed (a large building that can accommodate about 100 people, like an empty airplane hanger, with a concrete floor and no beds except for what you bring with you for bedding), I was trying to get some sleep, but people were snoring, going to the bathroom, and just moving here and there. Before long, word got out that I was a doctor and, when someone fell ill, I was asked to help. I tried to take a gentleman, who was having diarrhea, to the general hospital. We finally made it after overcoming several obstacles, such as the guard at the ashram not wanting to let us go since the hospital was supposed to be closed. After being persistent and finally getting to the hospital, I was soon put to work, not as a doctor but as a nurse! Since they were short on nurses, I was asked to be this gentleman's nurse, and I did this for a few days. However, much to my surprise, I was finally asked to stop. It seems I was trying to be in charge of his care and, foolishly, thought I knew more than the doctor in charge of the case did. The doctor in charge of this case happened to be a very smart, hardworking woman who is presently the acting medical director for the general hospital. What a humbling experience! I guess Swami knew that my ego needed deflating, and who is more expert at deflating one's ego than Sai Baba?

After returning home and processing all the events, I realized that, just because we do things differently in the USA, it does not mean that we are right or do things better than doctors in other countries. On the contrary, we have much to learn from foreign doctors who provide excellent and compassionate care.

Just to make sure that I did not forget the lessons learned while working as a nurse at the Sathya Sai General Hospital, I had the good fortune to work as a nurse again in 1997, this time in the USA. At that time, the registered nurses at Kaiser Permanente Hospital went on strike for a short period, and lucky doctors like myself had the wonderful opportunity to work as nurses during the strike. I believe I have always respected and appreciated the work nurses do, but it wasn't until I worked the night shift as a nurse in the emergency room at Kaiser that I fully appreciated just how hard they work and what very important work they do. Hopefully, I am now a more humble doctor.

Since this time, I have been back to India four times to see Sai Baba and work in His hospital. On each of these visits, I have had the good fortune to be able to work as a dermatologist at a medical camp in the ashram or at the clinic in the General Hospital. This has been a real blessing. Every time I return home, more of Sai Baba's infinite love and compassion has rubbed off on me. Swami advises doctors to, *Make love the capsule you offer to your patients. When a weak patient comes to you, do not be content with offering him glucose or some other thing. Give him the injection of Love. That will give him instant strength. Speak to him with love, offer medicines with love and keep him in good humor. That is the way to make him happy. Happiness is union with God. Anything you do with love will be rewarding.* On my most recent trip, I was allowed, once again, to work as a dermatologist in the General Hospital, along with the other doctors that work there on a regular basis. Where do you think they put me? The head doctor of the hospital had me work in a large spacious office that was meant for the medical director while he himself worked in another office down the hall, sharing a small room with another doctor. I thought that going from a rejected nurse to working in the medical director's office was pretty humorous. But the main thing is I realize that, when it comes to humility and curbing the ego, I still have a way to go.

Patience

One of the main influences Sai Baba has had on me is in helping me realize that, when I take care of a patient, I am being of service to God residing within that person. Knowing this has helped tremendously so that I am now more patient with my patients! I have an elderly patient, Mrs. T, who likes to talk about her family, especially her young grandchildren. Since her short term memory is not so good, she will usually tell me the same story about her grandchildren each time she comes in for a visit. She also likes to show me the same pictures. Mrs. T has no concept of time. She would talk to me indefinitely if I let her. In the past, this type of patient would make me extremely frustrated, especially if I was already behind schedule. I can still occasionally have this kind of reaction. However, most of the time now, as I enter the room, I smile, shake hands as I say hello and think, "Hello my dear Swami." This reminds me that I am really greeting the Lord and have a chance to serve Him. In Mrs. T's case, once this heart to heart connection was made, I was able to be fully present and focused on her, and we both felt more relaxed. We could enjoy the visit and still take care of her problem. When I take care of patients like Mrs. T, if I have to leave before they would like me to and I do so in a loving and sweet way, they do not seem to mind. Swami emphasizes that we use soft, loving speech with everyone, and I can tell you that patients really appreciate it when we talk to them in this manner.

Tolerance and Nonviolence

There are office visits when the patient I am taking care of is angry, rude, impatient, or downright hostile to me. I try and remember another teaching of Swami's, *To harm a person who harmed you is nothing great. Real greatness lies in loving the person who harmed you.* In most instances, if I can have the good sense to keep my heart open and continue to love them, before long their anger or impatience will melt away. Then, in some way, I will be able to help them. There are still some occasions when I respond to anger by getting angry, but I am getting so much better. Just recently, I had the good fortune to be tested to see if I was really putting this teaching into practice.

Mr. P is a burly Irishman with an unpleasant demeanor. I had not seen this patient before and was seeing him to give a second opinion about a chronic skin condition he had. I figured this visit was going to test my patience, when the receptionist warned me that Mr. P was already upset. He did not think that he should have to pay his $5 co-pay for the visit, since this visit was for a second opinion on a problem that he thought should have been taken care of by his previous doctor. As I walked into the exam room, I was met by a stern glare. Mr. P. sat on the exam table with his arms folded in front of him. I greeted him as I do all patients and tried to make a heart to heart connection with him. But, to my dismay, he proceeded to rant and rave about his previous medical care. He told me that he has no respect for any of the doctors who have cared for him and feels that no one who has seen him has given him good medical care. The visit lasted about twenty-five minutes, and most of this time was spent listening to Mr. P criticize all of his previous medical care. Several times during this visit I was tempted to put Mr. P in his place since some of his complaints were completely unreasonable. But for the most part, with Swami's help, I resisted. I was able to just let him vent and tried to understand why he was so angry. By the end of the visit, he had calmed down quite a bit, and we were able to agree on a treatment plan that he could understand and live with.

Judgments

I am not as judgmental about other doctors and patients as I used to be. When I used to hear about errors that other doctors made, or treatments they recommended that were different than what I would have prescribed, I would judge them harshly. Of course, I didn't say anything, but my thoughts were full of judgments. I now realize that most heath care providers try to do the best that they can, and certainly none of us are perfect.

I have been trying to see the good points in each person and not concentrate on his odd appearance or behavior. My patient, Sara, is a pleasant 21-year-old girl who works at the local health club. She has her ears pierced in several places, a ring in her eyebrow, tongue, and the area by the umbilicus (belly button). She came to see me to treat the piercing in her tongue which had caused an infection and a very thick scar called a keloid. The treatment of choice was to remove the ring to let the tongue heal up. Keeping the ring in place made the chance of healing much lower. However, she decided that she did not want to remove the ring in her tongue and wanted me to treat her with steroid injections in the tongue. I agreed to do this but warned her that the chance of success was low if she did not remove the ring. I must admit her choice of treatment seemed a bit odd to me and, in the past, I probably would have judged her to be some kind of oddball. I might even have talked to one of my fellow doctors or nurses later in the day about this weird patient and the fact that I thought that her choice to have her body pierced in so many odd places was ridiculous. Now, I try not to be judgmental or distracted by a person's physical appearance. The person may have his body pierced with rings in every conceivable location, he may be grossly overweight, underweight, or just plain filthy and smelly, but I try to see the good in him, reminding myself that I have this opportunity to serve God.

My interactions with nurses and receptionists in the office have changed for the better over the past few years too. If someone that I am working with doesn't seem to be doing his job properly, I will discuss this with him. However, in most cases, the negative things I notice are really minor in the whole scheme of things. Therefore, I try not to dwell on the negative traits but, instead, notice and compliment their good points. Swami has pointed out that it is not good to dwell on the negative traits in others but, rather, we should strive to see the good in others. If we dwell on the bad in others, we actually end up hurting ourselves. Swami says, *We become what we contemplate. By constant thought, an idea gets imprinted on our heart. When we fix our thoughts on the evil that others do, our mind gets polluted by the evil. When, on the contrary, we fix our mind on the virtues or well being of others, our mind is cleansed of wrong and entertains only good thoughts. No evil thought can penetrate the mind of a person wholly given to love and compassion.* He has also told us to be very critical when we evaluate our own actions but not to be harsh when we judge another person's actions. Of course, it is best not to be judgmental of the other person in the first place.

Understanding & Adjustment

Another teaching of Sai Baba's is *first understanding then adjustment.* This has helped me tremendously when dealing with patients who are angry and upset; Swami has said that, most of the time, we do just the opposite. For example, we react to a person's anger by telling them how unreasonable their anger is or by telling them what they should have done about the problem. We do this without first understanding exactly what the problem is or why they are so upset. In the past, when a patient was really upset about something, such as my being behind schedule, I would usually react immediately and, perhaps, make a judgment that the patient was being unreasonable.

Mrs. G, for example, arrived thirty-five minutes late for her appointment and then expected to be seen right after she arrived. In the past I may have reacted and said something like, "Mrs. G, my nurse tells me that you are upset because you had to wait twenty minutes to see me. I would just like to point out that it was you who arrived thirty-five minutes late. If, in fact, you had arrived on time, I would have been able to see you without a wait. However, since you were not here at your appointment time, and we had no idea whether or not you were going to come, I decided to see the next patient who had arrived on time." Of course this would justify my behavior but would do nothing to make my patient feel better. Besides, is it really so important that I was right and that I let her know she had no reason to complain? Now that I am trying to put Swami's teachings into practice, I will tell you how the visit actually went. "Hi, Mrs. G, my name is Dr. Phaneuf, I am sorry that I kept you waiting. Was there a problem with traffic in getting here? She responded, "Oh Dr. Phaneuf, thank you for seeing me when I arrived so late. This is my first time driving out here, and the traffic was bad, and I went to the wrong *Kaiser Clinic*; I thought that is where you were. I didn't mean to get upset, but I am supposed to pick up my daughter from day care in about thirty minutes, and I was afraid that I would get there late." Since I had listened to her, I could understand why she was upset. Now I was able to help her without getting upset back at her. Listening and understanding diffused and eventually eliminated her anger and impatience. If I am able to *first understand* what the problem is, then I can usually make an *adjustment* that will satisfy the patient and myself.

Guilt & Worry

I was raised in the Catholic faith. My mother was, and still is, a very devout Catholic. She is a shining example to me about how to be a good person and be of service to others. I was raised in a very loving and a very strict environment. Love of God and fear of sin was definitely emphasized in our home and at the Catholic school I attended. Over the years, I developed what many people refer to as Catholic guilt. This has remained with me on and off for most of my adult life. I have developed the very unhealthy habit of feeling guilty about things I have done wrong, or about things I could have done better. Consequently, I have wasted a lot of time and energy feeling guilty about the past. I also have worried too much about things that might happen in the future. The following two teachings of Sai Baba have helped me tremendously in this regard. *Worry is a waste of time and waste of time is waste of life. Whatever happens, say it is good for me.* I am really starting to believe this. Every mistake I make is a good learning experience. As long as I try not to make the same mistake again, there is no sense in rehashing the mistake over and over, feeling guilty, or whipping myself, so to speak. When I encounter a particularly stressful situation, I try to remember that this is a great opportunity to develop fortitude and, in fact, this seemingly bad situation is really good for me. I have also realized that when I dwell on mistakes I made in the past or worry about things that may happen in the future, I tend not to be present in the moment, since my attention and energy are diverted elsewhere. To overcome this tendency, I remind myself frequently of the following words of wisdom from Sai Baba:

Do not brood over the past. Past is past, forget it. Future is not certain. It is beyond your perception. So, live in the present; it is omnipresent. How? Past is in the present as the present is the result of past actions. Future is also in the present as it depends on the present actions. So, you should pay attention only to the present. Instead of giving importance to the ephemeral pleasures, you should follow the right path. That is all you are supposed to do now. But you are not doing what you are supposed to do. You simply brood over the past and worry about the future. In this way, you ignore the present. As a result, you are subjected to suffering. Why should you not derive happiness from the present state of affairs? Brooding over the past and worrying about the future are the main cause of man's suffering. Why do you think about the past? You treaded that path consciously. Then why do you look back? Be happy in the present. That is all you should aspire for. You may face many ordeals. But do not pay too much attention to them. Lead your life happily till the end.

Living in the present is wonderful. Previously, I had been so preoccupied with thinking about the past or the future that I was not able to focus and fully enjoy the present as much as I could have. I am extremely thankful to Swami for teaching me this very important concept.

Speak Obligingly

Another teaching of Swami's that has been of enormous benefit to me, and one that I have an opportunity to practice at least a dozen times each day is, *You can not always oblige, but you can always speak obligingly.* A patient may expect me to perform, for example, a cosmetic surgery for free even though it is a non-covered service. Although I cannot always oblige, if I explain why I cannot do what they request in a kind and caring way, then most patients can accept this without getting upset. Of course, if I am already connected heart to heart with the patient, they know that I am trying my best to help them, and they seem to be able to receive this news without "shooting the messenger."

Swami's Omnipresence

Lately, I am becoming more aware of Swami's omnipresence. At times, the realization of His omnipresence comes spontaneously, and I am aware of this on a deep experiential level. A good example of how some of this is starting to become spontaneous for me is the following recent patient encounter. I was actually finished seeing all of my afternoon patients. I had finished charting, going through lab and pathology reports, and had returned the necessary phone messages. I was ready to head out the door. My nurse then walked into my office to let me know that my last patient had arrived (thirty-five minutes late) and wanted to know if I could see her. In the past, I would have been aggravated and, even though I would see the patient, I would not be happy about it. I am sure most patients would pick up on this. In this case, I walked up to the front reception desk and looked at the patient who was waiting there. Then, something happened that really surprised me. When I gave the patient and her husband a warm smile, I felt love for them welling up inside me.

Prayer and Being an Instrument of God

As a dermatologist, I do surgical procedures such as removing skin cancers. Early in my career, before I knew about Swami, I would often worry about the way a complex surgery might heal - before, during, and after the procedure. It has been my practice, for the past few years, to say a prayer before I start an operation. I look at my hands just before I make the initial cut into the skin, and pray as follows: "Swami, these are your hands; please guide them to do this procedure." This gives me great confidence, and I feel that I do a better job when I let God guide my hands and help make decisions during the surgical procedure. When I pray to God in this manner and act with him as my inner guide, I feel that all of my actions will have the best possible outcome. I also tend to worry much less, since I also leave the outcome of the surgery to God and am not so attached or worried about the outcome.

Some of the results of the surgery that I have done have been nothing short of miraculous. Two cases come to mind. The first was a case that involved the surgical removal of a good size skin cancer on the right tip of the nose. The surgical defect (hole in the skin) was quite large, and I needed to rotate skin down from the upper part of the nose to fill in this defect. I had planned and planned for this procedure but, despite my best efforts, I was horrified when I realized that I had miscalculated the amount of tissue I needed to rotate down and I would come up short. I stretched the skin as tight as I could to get the surgical defect to close. However, when we have to stretch the skin this tight, there is a good chance that part of the skin flap may not survive and could turn gangrenous. I was extremely worried that part of the flap would not survive. Not only would the patient have a less than satisfactory cosmetic result, but this could also affect my reputation as a surgeon. I did a fair amount of worrying and a lot of praying. To my pleasant surprise, the surgery site healed so well that the scar was barely noticeable, and everyone was pleased with the final result.

Another case comes to mind where I removed a large skin cancer from the left side of the chin of a young man. This very large surgical defect also healed with hardly a noticeable scar. The divine energy that allows our bodies to heal the way they do after surgery, or after an injury, is absolutely miraculous. I am reminded of this on a daily basis when, post operatively, I am removing sutures from my patients and notice how well they are healing or when I see them several months or years after the surgical procedure.

Sometimes, if I feel a patient is open to it, I may advocate prayer. For instance, if they have a treatment resistant skin rash and all standard treatments have failed, I will still prescribe, or recommend, what would be considered conventional medical treatment. I then explain that, in my experience, a positive attitude and prayer may also be helpful. I cannot emphasize enough the power of love and prayer in the treatment of any condition. Love has the power to melt even God's heart, and anything is possible when we help another with love. Swami says, *Any incurable disease can be cured with love.*

Going with the Flow

In the past, when I worked in private practice, I had much more control over how I did things. I was the one who hired and supervised the nurses and receptionists who worked for me. Now that I work in a large group practice, I have no control over the nurses or receptionists, and I find that I have little or no say in how the office runs, with the exception of what I do when I am with the patient. This has certainly been a change and an adjustment for me. However, I realize that Swami's teaching, *Whatever happens, say it is good for me,* is actually true. He knew all along that one of my weak points was being inflexible.

Since working for Kaiser Permanente over the past four years, I have made a lot of improvement in this area. I am learning to "go with the flow." After many painful experiences, I have become much more flexible and less rigid.

For example, when I was in private practice, I usually had a nurse who assisted me with just about every procedure that I would do. Now, in my present job, I have had to learn to be more self-reliant. Since two to three doctors may share one medical assistant, I now do many surgical procedures by myself. However, I am able to have a medical assistant help me with surgical procedures when I feel that it is necessary. In addition, I apply dressings, give intramuscular shots and perform other tasks that, in the past, would have been done by my medical assistant or nurse. After much initial resistance, I have adjusted and actually enjoy this new way of doing things.

Another big advantage to working in a large group practice is that I interact with many other doctors and nurses who have different viewpoints. This presents a constant opportunity for friction. What a great way to expose my ego and self-interest!

For, only when these undesirable traits are exposed is it possible to examine them and let them go.

I am thankful to Sai Baba, beyond what words can express, to have been able to work in His hospital and serve Him by seeing His patients. After most overseas medical clinics, the doctors and nurses have received padnamaskar from Swami. This is a wonderful blessing, but I think Sai Baba is trying to wean us all off of this very joyous experience. Before the last overseas medical clinic in July 1999, Swami told the female medical doctors and nurses the following, *Being of service to your patients is My padnamaskar; I cannot give you anything higher than that.* This statement has made a very deep impression on me. I now realize that I do not have to go to India to see Swami in person, since I have the opportunity to be of service to God in each and every patient that I see in my clinic. I have learned by working in Sai Baba's hospital, and by reading His many discourses that, when I see a patient, I have the great opportunity to serve God who resides in that person. This has transformed the way I relate to my patients, to my medical practice, and to my life.

The Miracle of Prayer
Purnendu Dutta, M. D.

In 1950, I was thirteen years old and a ninth grade high school student in Calcutta. I clearly remember one day when our family doctor was drawing blood (200 ml) from my father and was throwing it in the drain as a treatment for his hypertension. With this sight, I fainted at my father's bedside. When I woke up, I was a totally different boy. A transformation had occurred in me. I felt a current flowing through me, and a divine presence commanding me to become a physician and help my father, who had hypertension and type 2 diabetes mellitus. I thought that there had to be a better way of treating him than letting out precious blood. This was the start of my dream of becoming a physician and a surgeon.

I knew that I had to overcome my fear of blood. My father and my uncle told me that, after taking a cold shower, I should worship the Sun God with proper rituals every morning at sunrise while offering flowers and Billapatra leaves and reciting sacred Sanskrit mantras. I did this for several years, and some wonderful things happened as a result. My grades at school improved beyond anyone's expectation, and my determination to become a doctor became even stronger.

My strong will and constant prayers helped me secure the highest qualifying scores for entry to medical school in Calcutta. As a medical student, I had the great desire to seek higher knowledge and training and to help the poor and underprivileged. These are all Sai principles, although I did not know about Him at this time. Towards the end of my medical school days, I heard about Lord Sai and His claim of being an incarnation of Shirdi Sai Baba. I made inquiries from family members and friends about this but found no proper information. I regret this very much, because I could have been further along on my journey. However, I was only twenty then.

After the completion of my postgraduate studies in surgery in Calcutta, I went to England for further training and became a fellow of the Royal College of Surgeons in England. My prayer and determination helped me get into the best training programs to gain more practical experience. The position of Surgical Registrar at the Royal Postgraduate Medical School in London became open and was advertised in the British Medical Journal. This was a very prestigious and difficult training position to obtain. As a matter of fact, my colleagues discouraged me from applying for the position, since the competition would be intense.

I was working in Manchester and wanted to see London. The interview for this position was on a Durga Puja Day. I thought this would be a perfect occasion to travel to London and see the Puja. When I was traveling from Manchester, I was constantly praying to Durga Mata, telling her that I would soon be coming to see her, and that she should be with me during the interview so that I could get the job. My prayers were heard. I was accepted for the post, even though there were many eligible local graduates competing with me. Before returning to Manchester, I enjoyed the Durga Puja celebration in London with my Indian friends. To this day no one, including myself, understands how I got that position. It could only be because of my prayers to Goddess Durga. It was this training, along with my contacts with the best doctors in the field of surgery, that helped me learn and advance in my field of work.

In 1968, I returned to Calcutta with great hopes and promises from the people at the top of the profession. They thought I would be able to find a position and practice what I had learned. However, I was greatly disappointed and constantly prayed for some opening in my field. During this fifteen-month period in India, a professor from Missouri, with whom I had worked at the Royal Postgraduate Medical School in London, invited me to come to the USA. He arranged for a research position for me at the University of Minnesota. This was the biggest 180-degree turn in my career. I never expected this to happen. Again, my prayers were answered. I embarked upon a very high level of training in surgical research. As a result of this, through another surgical colleague of mine with whom I had worked while in London in the same Postgraduate Medical School, I later obtained my current faculty position at the University at Buffalo School of Medicine. This is where I formed my roots and blossomed.

During the next fifteen years, I strove for excellence through prayers to God, superior training and continuing education. I believed in constant quality improvement and total quality management before they became the buzzwords in the industry. My area of interest was in gastrointestinal surgery. When the equipment became available, I taught myself gastrointestinal endoscopy and subsequently taught others. My fears in doing procedures were overcome by prayers before and during the cases, and I subsequently gave thanks to the Lord for avoiding catastrophes. I was performing procedures that others considered difficult. Since the procedures were new, I was without any formal training in this area and wondered who was actively guiding and helping me? Did I have a special talent or skill? I didn't think so. If I did, I would have been confident and probably not have required prayers.

Because of my ability to make correct diagnoses and perform surgery without difficulties, many of my colleagues became jealous and were extremely competitive with me. This led to many difficult times in my career until I was introduced to Baba in 1985. Finally, I realized who was behind all of my progress. I realized that Baba is God in every form, and that He had been the one guiding me all along. I am convinced that Baba is the supreme Lord whom I worshipped in the form of the Sun God and Goddess Durga in my early life. Now that I have found Him, I will hold on to Him forever.

I remember in 1985 at Baba's 60th birthday, the Williamsville Center in Buffalo arranged for an all-day open meeting, along with a great feast and scholarly talks from veteran Sai devotees from the Northeast region of the United States. Realizing who Baba was and what an opportunity I had missed for years, I was glad that I had finally found Him. I started attending regular bhajans and service activities at the center, enriching myself with Sai principles.

I went to Puttaparthi for the first time in 1987. My wife and my mother-in-law traveled with me. We arrived on Shivaratri day. During the morning darshan, after the auspicious night of Shivaratri, I was praying very hard that I would be seated in the front row to have a good darshan and possibly take padnamaskar from Baba. I received Baba's padnamaskar and blessing that very first morning. That same day, a miraculous thing happened. During the afternoon, I was wearing my sunglasses, and my regular prescription eyeglasses dropped out of my pocket. There were at least eight thousand people in the ashram compound. I thought the crowd would crush my eyeglasses into small pieces. I went to the registration office and asked for the lost and found box. There was nothing in it, but an elderly officer said, "Don't worry, come in the evening. Baba will find them for you." It was hard to believe; but nevertheless, it was a comforting statement. I am severely myopic and did not want to ruin my future darshans with blurred vision. Sure enough, with Baba's grace, I found the pair of eyeglasses in the lost and found box and, like a fool, I checked that they had my prescription in them and that they were free from scratches. My wife and my mother-in-law were astonished with this miracle. Our stay was most enjoyable, and my belief and faith in Baba was greatly strengthened.

I visited Puttaparthi again in 1989. This time I was alone. All my time was spent in prayer, meditation, darshan and contemplation. During the first morning darshan, I was seated in the third row. While Baba took the letters I offered Him, I asked Him for "Ashirvad" (blessing). Baba raised His hand and looked straight into my eyes uttering, *Ashirvad.* My heart filled with joy, and my eyes with tears. During the afternoon darshan, on the day before I was returning home, a seva dal allowed me to sit in the front on the main entranceway to the mandir compound. This was not a usual seating area, but they allowed this because of the large crowd on that day in December. Baba gave His darshan and, as usual, walked past. After some time, for reasons unknown, He came back and stood in front of me at a distance of five or six feet. He never spoke a word with anyone, but I had several periods of eye contact with Him. He stood there for more than fifteen minutes and was gesturing with His hands while listening to the bhajans in the background. I had the unique opportunity of worshipping Him quietly. It felt like the darshan was just for me. I came home with my heart full of joy and my mind highly charged with spirituality.

Ever since, I have felt Baba's presence and guidance in everything I do. I seek His permission and help all the time. I am not afraid of treating seriously ill patients knowing that Baba, the great beacon and guide, will be with me, giving me courage and inspiration. I believe that Baba will help me improve my skill in overcoming all adverse situations in my practice of medicine and surgery.

There are many instances in my practice where extremely difficult situations were overcome by some inexplicable supernatural intervention. I attribute this to Baba. To me, God is Baba and Baba is God. It is all Baba's leela. All of the following cases demonstrate the active help Baba has given me over the years.

Case 1: Multiple Endocrine Tumors
There was a middle-aged man whom I started to treat for peptic ulcer disease. He soon developed a tumor in his parathyroid gland with high calcium level in his blood. I removed the tumor from his neck with great success. The ulcer disease in his stomach deteriorated and, soon, he was diagnosed to have tumors in his pancreas, which were responsible for increased acid production from his stomach and ulcer formation. He needed a total removal of his stomach, a formidable undertaking. He was also anemic with increased risk from surgery. Other surgeons were skeptical about his surgery. I presented the case before a panel of physicians and surgeons. The consensus was to treat him medically and not to take undue surgical risk. At this point, I was very disheartened and disappointed that the patient would have to suffer tremendously for the rest of his life. I started praying to Baba for help and gained courage to do the right thing, which was surgery. I spent several sleepless nights at the hospital taking care of this sick man and constantly praying for his life. My prayers were answered, and he survived with a great result. In subsequent years, he developed chronic renal failure requiring hemodialysis. However, he lived longer than anyone had expected. Without Baba's help and guidance, I could not have helped this man.

Case 2: Cancer of Stomach, Colon and Pancreas
This was the case of a middle-aged man who was the hospital barber where I worked. Like most barbers, this man was very friendly and was liked by everyone. He had a small shop at the basement of the hospital. The hospital staff and patients were his

clients. One day, the chief of the urology department called to tell me that the barber, who was his friend, was diagnosed with advanced cancer of the abdomen and that his doctors felt that nothing could be done for him. He was suffering greatly with pain and was unable to eat properly. I felt very sorry for the barber who was left to undergo the natural course of the dreadful disease. My urologist friend was hoping that I would be able to help. I started praying hard to Baba to give me some insight into this patient's problem. I accepted the patient for evaluation first and confirmed the diagnosis of cancer of the stomach, which may have spread to the surrounding organs. CT scan was not available at that time. After more prayers to Baba, I gathered courage and explained to the family that I would explore the patient's abdomen, hoping that I would be able to do something to help him. During surgery, I found that the tumor had invaded part of the adjoining colon and the tail and body of the pancreas. I had never before had any experience of doing an en block resection surgery of this magnitude. I almost gave up. I prayed intensely to Baba for help and guidance. Suddenly, I felt some strength, and I realized that this operation was the only chance that this man had for any kind of relief of symptoms. I removed most of his stomach, part of his colon and part of his pancreas in one block. This was not a curative operation by any means. At best it was palliative. The man, however, was able to eat and gain weight and was free of pain. He lived for eighteen months following surgery and was able to take care of his family duties before passing away peacefully. Only Baba's help had made this possible. If I had had this patient prior to my introduction to Baba, I would not have ventured into this risky surgical procedure.

Case 3: Upper Gastrointestinal Bleeding

A young African American woman in her late twenties was brought to the emergency room with massive upper gastrointestinal bleeding. I was on call, and people knew of my skills with endoscopy. After initial resuscitation, requiring blood transfusion, I looked into her esophagus and stomach with the endoscope. She was bleeding from superficial ulcerations in her stomach. She also had prominent esophageal varices, but they were not bleeding. I treated her with conservative measures. She stopped bleeding and promptly recovered. After five days, she re-bled massively. On scoping again, I found that her ulcers were not bleeding at this time, but there was massive bleeding from the esophageal varices, which are cherry-like blood vessels in the lower esophagus. I treated her with conservative measures of blood transfusion and intravenous pitressin drip. She continued to bleed. I was spending nights at the hospital trying to resuscitate her. She was in the intensive care unit for the whole time and was being fed intravenously with nutrients. By this time, she had received many units of transfusion of blood and various blood products. She was a very poor risk for surgery. I consulted with some other surgical colleagues of mine. Everyone suggested conservative medical management. I felt that this woman's life was threatened. She was the mother of two very young children. I prayed to Baba for help. I thought that surgery, although extremely risky, was her only way out of trouble. As she was going downhill, I intensified my prayers. Baba eventually gave me the courage to take her into surgery. This time, I needed to create a bypass between her portal and systemic venous systems, a really major undertaking and a great risk after so much bleeding. Upon exploration, I could not find a portal vein as there was a cavernous malformation of the portal system. I ended up doing a mesocaval shunt operation with an 'H' graft with a synthetic material called Gortex. This involved connecting two large veins with this artificial tube enabling blood to flow, thereby bypassing the obstruction. During the whole procedure I was silently praying, asking for some light into this difficult situation. Baba was kind enough to help me. The patient survived and is doing well eighteen years later. The family wants to give the credit to me, but I have been successful in convincing them that it was God who saved her life.

Case 4: Diabetic Cellulitis and Gangrene of Both Hands and Forearms

This was an obese woman in her late forties. She came to the hospital with severely swollen hands and forearms with gangrenous areas on both sides. She was a severe diabetic with poor control of her blood sugar and poor general hygiene. At times, we thought that she might end up losing both her hands. I was on call. My first reaction was, "Baba, why me?" In this litigious society, the last thing I wanted was a case where the patient had the real potential of losing both hands. However, I had sympathy for this woman as she begged me to do my best. I consulted with several of my colleagues who expressed the opinion that this woman would most likely lose her hands. I started to pray to Baba and explained all the risks to the patient and her husband. They seemed to have understood the dangers of this advanced disease.

I first controlled her blood sugar with careful titration of insulin. Then I took her to surgery. I prayed to Baba for His guidance in recognizing the dead tissue versus the viable one so that I might remove only what was dead. Under general anesthesia, I removed all the dead tissue from her hands and forearms. Then I incised all fascial compartments and left all wounds open to drain freely. In subsequent discussions at clinical conferences, other doctors expressed that they would have removed more tissue, which would have eventually led to amputations. During the weeks that followed, I prayed constantly to Baba for her healing. In about three months, with special care and some skin grafting, she managed to keep both of her hands. Some stiffness of the fingers developed, but she learned to live with it. This was Baba's miracle. I would not have had the courage to do such conservative treatment, risking profound sepsis and further complications, if it was not for my deep faith in Baba and the power of prayer.

Case 5: Diabetic Gangrene of Both Feet

Soon after the preceding case, in a different hospital, an elderly African American woman from a poor socio-economic background was admitted under my care. I felt that God had sent this patient along to me because of my experience with the other case. She had diabetic gangrene of both feet, and her doctors recommended amputation of her legs. I presented her in our clinical conference. All the doctors recommended amputation. I prayed to Baba for this woman and asked Him to save her legs and feet. I applied the same principles learned from my previous case. I controlled her diabetes, debrided dead tissue and made multiple incisions in the feet to promote proper drainage of infected exudates. It worked in our favor again, but only because of a lot of prayers. The lady was able to walk out of the hospital after four months. During her hospital stay, I had to constantly fight with the utilization review department and the HMO because of her long stay; but in the end, I was successful in justifying her time in the hospital. If I had performed amputation, her hospital stay would have been much shorter, which the HMO would have liked. It was very satisfying for me to see her, once again, walk on her own feet. This patient's legs were saved because Baba heard my prayers.

Case 6: Toxic Megacolon with Perforations

A middle-aged woman was brought into the hospital with severe abdominal pain and distention. She was found to have bowel perforation, which required immediate surgery. She was in septic shock. I was on call that night. I took her to surgery after initial resuscitation. Upon opening the belly I saw that most of her colon was necrotic. Stool was leaking freely from multiple areas in the colon into the peritoneal cavity. There was stool all over the peritoneal cavity. With this amount of peritoneal contamination with fecal matter and with septic shock, hardly anyone survives. Her condition deteriorated. The anesthesiologist was worried about her vital signs. I had to hurry. I prayed silently, as best as I could, for her life. I asked Baba to guide me during the procedure in every step. In order to clean the fecal matter, I washed the entire abdominal cavity with warm saline and made multiple openings into the large bowel at the necrotic sites. Then I fixed those openings to holes made in the abdominal wall; these corresponded with those openings in the bowel. This way, fecal matter could come out directly through multiple openings to the outside without further soiling of the peritoneal cavity. I left multiple drains in the peritoneal cavity for any exudate to come out freely. I discussed the case in our clinical conference. No one in the hospital expected her to survive. But my prayers were heard. She recovered in ten days and went home. Several weeks later, I was able to remove her diseased large bowel and put it together for bowel movement to occur in the normal way. I feel strongly that, without Baba's help, the outcome would have been different.

In all these cases, I had to turn to Baba for help as these situations were extremely difficult. I needed courage and guidance in order to avoid making a mistake. It is my firm belief that without Baba's help, I would not have ventured into such risky treatments and, certainly, would not have been successful. It is only Baba who can perform miracles. We, as physicians, are Baba's instruments in healing patients. To us, a favorable outcome in the face of all hazards is Sai's grace. If we are the treating physicians, and we have prayed to Baba for help, we have to accept that it was Baba's miracles that saved the patients when the odds were against them.

I have always believed in God and prayed to Him. After I came to know Lord Sai deeply, in 1985, I realized that Baba is the Supreme Lord. All forms of God are His. Since then, I only pray to Baba. Before my closeness to Baba was developed, I depended more on my medical and technical knowledge than on the power of prayer in my practice of medicine and surgery. But after Baba came into my life, I have dedicated everything to Him. I believe I am His instrument. Because I dedicate the results to Him all the time, I have less stress and fear. I ask Him to give me the intelligence and skill to perform the duties assigned by Him to me. He has enhanced my ability to serve my patients effectively, successfully, and with deep concentration. He has given me the courage and confidence in treating difficult surgical conditions. I look upon myself as a servant carrying out His wishes. In this way, He is always responsible and will always do the right thing. I have become extremely humble since coming to Baba. I no longer like to take credit for any of the successes in my practice.

As a Sai physician, I know I must be very knowledgeable and pay a lot of attention to detail, because Baba is a very strict disciplinarian. He takes no short cuts and is extremely thorough in everything He does. Like Baba, I must also be full of love and compassion and see Sai in all my patients. Under all circumstances, I must be eager to help all those in distress. As a Sai physician, I must have the highest standard of morals and professional conduct and follow all the rules and standards of good practice. I must take care of my own health in order to remain physically fit to take care of others at all times of the day or night. It is most important that I remember that my acquired knowledge is minuscule in comparison to the vast universal wisdom of Sai. For this reason, I constantly meditate and pray for Lord Sai to guide and help me in all the difficult situations during the treatment of patients.

Becoming a physician has given me the unique opportunity to serve the sick and the needy. I now feel when I treat my patients that I am in Baba's service. I offer my pranams to Lord Sai for His constant guidance and His healing miracles in my medical practice.

There should be a harmonious blend of religion, philosophy and art for man to live healthily in the world. In this context, religion means the religion of love. This is the only religion in the world. There is only one caste, the caste of humanity. One should cultivate human values for healthy living. This calls for harmony of thought, words and deed. When you cultivate this harmony, you will be free from desires and fears.

Sathya Sai Baba
Sanathana Sarathi, Vol. 36 #3, March 1993

The Unseen Hand of God

Dr. Sara Pavan, M.B.B.S. (Cey), F.R.C.A. (Eng)

It is with humility and gratitude to my Beloved Master, Bhagavan Sri Sathya Sai Baba, that I take on the task of conveying the subtlety and profundity of some of my personal experiences which, without His grace, would have been extremely difficult. I dedicate this modest contribution to the infinitely loving and grace bestowing Lord, my loving Swami, Sri Sathya Sai Baba, who has stood by me and lent me His unseen hand many a time.

I was born in Malaysia. When World War II ended, my family moved to Ceylon, now Sri Lanka, where I completed my education and qualified as a medical doctor in 1962. After getting married in 1965, my wife, also a doctor, and I left for Singapore where the Singapore Health Department gave us a three-year contract. We had no choice in our postings. I was posted to Anesthesia, a specialty I disliked very much and had tried to avoid in the past. My interest at the time was in surgery, and I was, therefore, studying for the Surgery Part I examination. With the East African Asians flooding into the United Kingdom in 1967, my British passport became a worthless document. I got marooned in Singapore as a "stateless" person. Because of this situation, my superior, the chief anesthetist, urged me to pursue my career in Anesthesia, assuring me that this could be my solution. He felt it could be my international passport to success and resolve my stateless situation. So I closed my anatomy books and started studying Pharmacology and, by God's grace, passed the Australian Anesthesia Part I examination in August 1967. The prospect became grim when the Singapore government was unwilling to extend our contract. However, the unseen hand of God resolved my stateless dilemma by having the Australian government grant us permanent migration. Because I had a country that would accept me as a resident, overnight my British passport became a valid document for travel to Britain! We had the choice between going to Australia or the UK, but since training prospects in Britain were better at the time, we proceeded to the UK. I completed my specialization as a Fellow of the Faculty of Anesthetists of the Royal College of Surgeons in January 1969. I worked as Consultant Anesthetist in the UK until

1972, then in New Zealand for three years before settling in Sydney in 1975.

I was born in a modest middle-class Hindu family and joined in family prayers and temple visits. When I was growing up these activities did not appeal to me, because they appeared as mere routine. However, I did pray to God to help me pass my examinations. After I became a student of modern science and medicine, living mostly in the west, I no longer thought about God. Although my life was riddled with adversities, success came my way. With hindsight, it was easy to recognize the hand of God that led me to specialize in Anesthesia, for this indeed turned out to be my international passport to success. Totally oblivious to God, I continued my life as a rationalist and sought higher professional and worldly attainments. I ceased seeking places of worship or praying to God like those around me. I even "played God" when the mantle of decision-making fell on my head as to which patient should be taken off the life support system. I felt I was the doer and that I knew what I was doing. I had a cynical outlook towards religious people in society, even calling them weak minded. I had come across individuals who, although garbed in saffron, were deceiving naïve people. This made me suspicious of all men in ochre robes.

I first heard about Sai Baba in 1968 from an old school teacher of mine and again in 1972 from a doctor friend of my wife. I not only totally rejected but also conspicuously condemned Sai Baba. One day, while playing golf along with some elite members of New Zealand society, I had an extraordinary experience. I "saw" a review of my life flash across my mental screen. I "saw" my early years where, until I secured a place in medical school, I could not even afford a pair of decent shoes. Life was riddled with disappointments, adversities, and financial difficulties. It was this experience that enabled me to acknowledge the unseen hand of God. I knew that He had safely brought my wife and me ashore through the rough uncharted waters of life. I saw that every setback had laid the unseen foundation for greater success. We were granted even more than we ever bargained for. With this sudden realization in 1974, I began earnestly to seek the unseen One but certainly not Sai Baba.

In my search for this invisible hand of God that had protected and guided me all along, I began sifting through the lives and messages of Sri Ramakrishna, Swami Vivekananda, Paramahamsa Yogananda, Ramana Maharshi and Sri Aurobindo. I also got initiated into Maharishi Mahesh Yogi's technique of Transcendental Meditation. Having exhausted these avenues without satisfaction, my search turned towards Sai Baba. I began reading about this God man with deep interest. On March 30, 1980, He appeared to me in a dream. I had smoked about thirty cigarettes a day for twenty-five years and was deeply addicted to it. After this dream, my addiction ceased, and I no longer had an urge to smoke. In the two months that followed, I had more dreams and experiences that led me to become a teetotaler and vegetarian as well. This was after being a heavy smoker, above average social drinker, and enjoying all kinds of non-vegetarian food. I wondered what Sai Baba had done to my inner chemistry to bring about this mysterious transformation. The fact that I moved away from these things so thoroughly, in the midst of living an affluent western lifestyle, could not be considered anything but a miracle. Since my first dream of Sai Baba, I also had the mystical experience of being engulfed, every waking hour, by the smell of jasmine. This continued until we visited Him in Prasanthi Nilayam for the first time in December 1980. From that point on, I became fully committed to spiritual life.

Our first visit to Sai Baba in December 1977 was unexpected. We were visiting tourist sites in India. When we were in Bangalore, we became curious to see Sai Baba. With the persistence of our taxi driver, we changed our program and went to Whitefield where Baba was at the time. Even though I witnessed Baba materializing vibhuti for a devotee right in front of me, it had no impact on me. It was only when we visited Him in Prasanthi Nilayam in December 1980 that our hearts overflowed with love and devotion. We were blessed with two consecutive interviews. Our first experience, face-to-face with Baba, was one of tremendous emotional upheaval, when sublime forces from deep within burst out, releasing our innermost feelings with copious tears. It was like a long-lost child reuniting with its mother. Very little conversation was possible, and Swami asked us to come again for another interview the following morning. Swami gave us a lot of attention and told us many things about our past, what we were supposed to do for the present, and He also revealed His future plans for us. He told us that in ten years we would live with Him, and that He would build a super specialty hospital in Puttaparthi where I would serve Him as an Anesthetist. December 29, 1980 was the momentous day when Swami gave us a glimpse into the future plan for Puttaparthi, then a remote hamlet in India. No one would have believed at the time that a high-tech hospital in Puttaparthi could ever be a reality.

Since then, we visited Baba every year and were blessed with many personal interviews. By His grace, we have directly experienced that Baba is aware of everything. He can intervene in any situation, distance and time being no limitation. We have also seen His invisible hand at work. We have experienced His divine presence many a time, in response to our heartfelt call, and witnessed miraculous outcomes in hopeless situations through His timely intervention. We have experienced and witnessed Sai miracles of all kinds, but I am limiting them to medically oriented ones for this book. Our first such experience was with Rev. Ted Mulvehill, a Catholic priest from South Australia, who was visiting Baba's ashram during our visit in December 1982.

Mysterious Fits Cured

December 19, 1982 was an eventful and unforgettable day for us. Baba had blessed our family with an interview in the morning and materialized for me a silver ring with His head and shoulders on solid gold relief. Before we left the interview room, He also gave us plenty of vibhuti packets. There were so many devotees from Australia that year, and they appeared to outnumber the rest of the foreigners. It seemed it would be an Australian Christmas. Arthur Hillcoat, an Australian devotee and presently a Central Coordinator in the Sai Organization, was waiting for us at the gate of the darshan ground. As soon as we came out of the interview room, Arthur whisked my wife and me away to attend to Rev. Ted Mulvehill, a Catholic priest from Adelaide, who was unconscious and had been having fits for over an hour.

As we rushed to Ted's room, we were vaguely briefed about his condition. Neither of us is a Neurologist nor can claim to have specialist knowledge to diagnose accurately and treat such a condition. We learned from a young doctor, who had accompanied Ted, that he had been fully examined at Flynders Institute in Adelaide, and his fits fell neither into the usual categories of epilepsy nor responded to conventional medication. His attacks had been irregular and unpredictable and could only be temporarily stopped by intravenous Valium. There was no known prophylaxis that would help Ted. We were fresh from the interview room armed only with Baba's vibhuti and faith in Him alone.

When we arrived in Ted's room, we found him unconscious and having generalized fits and lying on the floor with his eyes rolled up and his tongue protruding to one side. He was not responding to his name. The young doctor had brought with him intravenous Valium, but this time, even the Valium was ineffective and no one knew what to do. I thought, "If Flynders Institute, a teaching hospital in Australia with all its high powered investigations, could not sort this out and find an effective cure for Ted, what chance do we have in Prasanthi Nilayam?" We had only "Dr. God," our beloved Baba, at our disposal, and we were entirely at His mercy. We prayed for Swami's help and applied vibhuti to Ted's forehead, chest, and upper limbs, as well as put a pinch of it on his tongue. There was no immediate change. Arthur happened to see my shining ring and asked me if Baba had materialized it for me in the interview. When I concurred, Arthur suggested that I place the ring on Ted's forehead and continue praying. The response was immediate. Ted rolled his eyes towards me and in slurry words said, "Is that you Sara? Thank you so much." Ted recovered fully and was given the important role of narrator in the Christmas program. He had no further attacks while in Prasanthi Nilayam. I have kept in touch with

Rev. Ted Mulvehill since then, and he always tells me with delight that December 19, 1982 was his last seizure. Almost eighteen years have rolled by, and Ted's mysterious fits had been permanently cured by Swami's grace.

From the "Sai Pharmacy"

It was during this same visit that we were blessed with another interview. The world famous sitar maestro, Pandit Ravi Shankar, sat immediately in front of Sai Baba. My wife and I were seated on either side at Swami's feet. For a couple of minutes Swami spoke in Hindi with the great musician in Hindi. The only English word I heard was "gastric." During the conversation, Swami pointed towards his stomach. All of a sudden, Swami waved His right hand in a circle and clenched His fist as He stopped the motion. He turned towards me first and opened His hand, and there were three large white tablets. Swami, with His eyes sparkling said to me, *From the Sai Pharmacy.* He turned towards my wife and repeated the same words as He showed the tablets to her as well. Then, He broke the tablets into halves and gave the six halves to Pandit Ravi Shankar and asked him to take one-half three times a day for two days and reassured him that all would be well.

I have heard that Baba has materialized various tablets, capsules, and bottles of eye drops. I know first hand of an instance where Baba had materialized surgical instruments and performed surgery on the eye of a blind young man from the UK, restoring his eyesight. Then to complete His divine healing process, He produced a bottle of eye drops with a wave of His hand. Countless are the instances of miracle cures. How and why He does all this is beyond our understanding. We witness these miracles with great awe and experience His divinity in His multifarious manifestations.

Cardiac Arrest

Since the Mulvehill episode, I have learned to call on Swami whenever I am faced with a dire emergency. My faith was further reinforced by similar experiences of devotees who had prayed for

Swami to intercede in desperate situations. I had no doubt that Swami had unlimited powers to intercede, that such powers were inscrutable, and that to Him distance was no barrier at all. One day, I had an elderly Chinese gentleman, a diabetic and hypertensive, anesthetized for excision and reconstructive plastic surgery for malignant melanoma on his face. Hardly had the operation commenced when I had to go to the adjoining room to administer anesthetic for an emergency Cesarean section, leaving this patient in the care of a junior resident. As soon as the baby was delivered and things were on course in the second operating room, I wandered into the first room to check if all was well. The first thing I saw was the flat ECG trace. The face looked deathly pale and I alerted everybody. I could not feel the carotid pulse nor could the surgeon feel the femoral pulse. The scrub sister removed her gloves and ran out for the defibrillator. I thought this was too much for me to cope with, especially with the Cesarean patient still on the table. After a few seconds of External Cardiac Massage, I paused for a moment and, placing my golden Baba ring over the patient's heart, I prayed for help. Considering the age and the pre-existing medical condition I felt that, even if the resuscitation was successful, this patient was going to need intravenous infusion of several life support drugs. Above all, he would need time to recover from possible damage to the vital organs, especially the kidney and brain.

With my eyes closed I prayed to Swami, "Please don't make this a long struggle for all of us and then leave the patient like a vegetable. Please help Swami." When I opened my eyes, I was awe-struck to see the face flushed and color improving. I could now feel the carotid pulse and the ECG tracing reappeared even without any drug having been given to revive the patient. Although the blood pressure was still low, the patient's color continued to improve. I had no words to explain what had happened to the patient, and I was unconcerned about others in the room making their own conclusion. I silently thanked my beloved Swami and reassured the surgeon that we were back on track and that he should proceed with the operation.

Anesthetized Patient Has a Bird's Eye View

In the eighties, on some free weekends, I would drive to the outback country towns in New South Wales to meet people, talk of my experiences, show videos and films of Swami, and provide books and tapes. On one such trip, a lady came up to me at the end of my talk and asked me if I would arrange for a surgeon in Sydney to operate on her varicose veins and if I would give her the anesthetic myself. Since there was a waiting list in the public hospital, it was easier for me to arrange for her to have this done in a private hospital where I happened to work with a reputed surgeon. Melanie was admitted on a Sunday and scheduled for surgery the next day. She was a slim built and very pleasant lady. I did a pre-operative check the night before, and she was fine. She was very relaxed and wanted to know more about Sai Baba. I spent a further twenty minutes talking with her. She preferred not to have any pre-medication for the anesthetic.

She was first on the list the next morning and was very relaxed. After so many years of practice and faith in Swami, I endeavor to be as practical and simple as possible, both in my approach to the patient and the anesthetic technique, following the maxim, "KISS", meaning **K**eep **I**t **S**hort & **S**imple. I kept her anesthetic as simple as possible—induced with Thiopentone and maintained anesthesia with Oxygen, Nitrous Oxide and Halothane via mask secured by a harness which allowed her to breath effortlessly. The operation took just over half an hour. Her anesthetic was maintained at a moderately deep level with 2% Halothane. A local doctor, whom Melanie had never seen before, came to assist the surgeon, and he arrived after Melanie was anesthetized. In the post-operative room, she recovered quickly without any ill effect, had no pain whatsoever and did not need any analgesia even though she had no analgesic drug pre-operatively or during surgery. She was quite excited and told the recovery staff her incredible experience under anesthesia, which she couldn't wait to tell me.

"As soon as you had injected the anesthetic I began to leave my body and drift upwards, piercing through the overhead operating light and perched myself in one corner of the ceiling. I had a bird's eye view of what was going on below. You had fastened a black mask over my face and connected it to a tubing and bag. They tilted my body slightly to a side, painted my legs and covered my body with green drapes. The surgeon walked in through the side door of the room. A short stubby man followed him. I could see his beard sticking outside his mask. Both were gowned and gloved. Who was he? I had never seen him before." I told Melanie that he was a GP who came to assist with the operation.

Melanie described the operation quite vividly. By now I was ready to face some embarrassment when she looked at me smiling and said, "I saw you seated comfortably and reading a magazine." I defended myself saying, "Didn't you see my left hand on your pulse continuously taking care of you?" "I know," she continued, "I was not afraid. The real surprise, you know, was that Sai Baba was standing close to the surgeon and directing him, and there was a glow over the surgeon's sleeves." This last observation stirred my gratitude and devotion to our omnipresent and omnipotent Sai. Melanie had no pain, even though she had no narcotic whatsoever. Her recovery was smooth and speedy.

In an out-of-body experience, an individual sees one's own body from a distance, usually hovering over the body and witnessing things happening in its surroundings. But awareness during anesthesia is mostly due to inadequate anesthetic, causing the patient to be awake and know what is happening. Three decades ago, the phenomenon of awareness during anesthesia came to the fore and extensive research had been done on this subject. Irrespective of the depth of anesthesia, a few in a million, upon recovery, experience awareness with recall of some incident or conversation in the operating room. After some thirty-five years of full time anesthetic practice and giving tens of thousands of anesthetics, this is the first and only instance I have encountered of an out-of-body experience under anesthesia. It is an extremely rare occurrence.

We may have progressed by leaps and bounds in science and technology, but we also appear to have regressed in inverse proportion from the holistic and spiritual approach. These days psychology, the science of mind and emotions, and the art of counseling and reassuring patients seem totally neglected in both undergraduate and even postgraduate training. Very few even care to remember that there is a person with feelings in the body. We have the scientific knowledge but lack an understanding heart. The psychic domain of emotion, fear and anxiety respond best to compassion, love and reassurance. Medication for anxiety has limitations too. Winning the patient's confidence is the best way to relieve anxiety.

Fear of death under anesthesia is a powerful negative emotion. Both anesthetists and surgeons must consider it their duty to tackle this problem in a holistic way. Modern doctors find it almost impossible to communicate with patients in a compassionate and loving way, especially to integrate spirituality with medicine by bringing God and His boundless grace into the picture. This is a vital link which is sadly missing. The workload is also heavy in most hospitals. It is not always possible to do such counseling, especially in emergency situations, even if the doctor is endowed with these skills. However, some improvements in the work schedule, better staffing, and greater holistic awareness among all health care workers may improve this situation.

A wide section of the medical profession would be cynical, or even hostile, to the suggestion that there is an aspect of the mind, deep and inscrutable, that has a spiritual or psychic dimension and could explain the source of fear or other negative stress responses. Unless we broaden our outlook and spiritual vista, we cannot understand the subjective and psychic nature of a patient's perceptions. We need to understand and accept even out-of-body experiences such as the one Melanie had. Awareness is paradigmatic. The time is fast approaching for the clinician to look beyond his limited objective vision and try to understand the innermost feelings of another individual. Dr. MacFarland Burnett, a Nobel Prize winning microbiologist from Australia, once said, "Viruses are a spectrum of biological patterns." Why should it then be difficult for us to understand that humanity is a spectrum of spiritual patterns? The surgical team, which includes an anesthetist, must manifest self-confidence and beget the same in all their patients. We must show openness with patients and their next of kin and instill in them hope where there is despair.

During my early years in practice in Anesthesia and Intensive Care, I had neither interest nor understanding of the many factors behind pain, fear and emotion, which were lumped together as surgical or hospital stress. My so-called rational and mechanistic view limited my practice to scientific usage of drugs and technology without a deeper understanding of the human personality. I got elated with achievements and became dejected when things went wrong. It never occurred to me that there was something beyond me that had brought about these results. Since my search into the meaning of life began in earnest in the mid seventies, and especially after experiencing Baba's omnipresence, omnipotence and His unseen hand at work, my whole attitude towards patients and clinical situations has steadily changed. I feel His presence most of the time and consciously work in His presence. Whenever I overcome difficult situations, I always thank Him for His help. Since I became a devotee of Sai Baba, my attitude toward work has changed drastically. I have no difficulty relating to all patients alike—rich or poor, private or public—whereas in the past, I had given more attention to private and wealthy patients. Since 1993, I am blessed to be able to serve as honorary anesthetist in Baba's world famous hospital, the Sri Sathya Sai Institute of Higher Medical Sciences, at His abode in Prasanthi Nilayam. It is entirely voluntary on my part, and I have no anxieties about money matters or differential considerations between poor peasants, wealthy landlords and businessmen, or the so-called VIPs. At both the Sri Sathya Sai Institute of Higher Medical Sciences and the Sathya Sai General Hospital, all patients are treated entirely fee.

A Miraculous Cure with Vibhuti

Another phenomenal experience was with Rev. Ted Noffs, Pastor of the Wayside Chapel, who was stricken with a massive cerebral hemorrhage in February 1987. He was unconscious and fighting for his life when he was admitted into the Intensive Care

Unit. This was at St. Vincent's Hospital, one of the foremost teaching hospitals in Sydney. After three days, Ted's condition was so poor that the doctors abandoned all hope for his survival and informed the family that Ted would not even last a few hours. Still in a coma, he was breathing oxygen via a clear plastic facial mask. Having known me very well for a few years, as well as knowing about some of Sai Baba's miraculous cures, the family decided, as a last resort, to accept a packet of Baba's vibhuti. I suggested that they apply some to Ted's forehead, neck and chest, as well as put a pinch of it on his lips. After all, what did they have to lose, they queried. "No sooner had the vibhuti touched Ted's lips," said Mrs. Noffs, "when I saw him come alive. His face turned bright and the lips became flushed. The vibhuti also multiplied so profusely that it not only started filling the mask, but also started clogging the oxygen inlet. We were very worried that the nurses on duty might witness this, so we quickly lifted the mask and wiped the ash away with a prayer of thanks to Sai Baba." Although Ted Noffs had not recovered fully, he lived for seven more years.

Control Over Drug Action—Distance No Barrier

The bedside phone rang at 3 a.m. on a winter night. I was called in to anesthetize a woman who had twins in fetal distress and required an urgent Cesarean section. It happened to be her first pregnancy, and she looked forward to having these two precious infants. The hospital was fifteen minutes away by car, and the obstetrician asked me to go straight to the operating suite on the sixth floor. After changing my apparel, I rushed into the operating room. The patient was already on the operating table with the midwife monitoring the fetal heart. The OT sister was scrubbing up, and a junior nurse was setting up two trolleys for resuscitation of the infants. Straight away, I started drawing up drugs in syringes. The obstetrician came towards me and told me that the cervix was fully dilated and that he would attempt to deliver the fetuses vaginally.

I often use different size syringes for different drugs to avoid any mix up, especially so in very urgent Cesareans. In such instances, writing labels and sticking them to syringes can cause some delay. I limit myself to three syringes only—10 ml for Thiopentone with Atropine for speedy induction, 2 ml syringe for Suxamethonium (quick and short acting muscle relaxant) for speedy endotracheal intubation and 5ml syringe for Vecuronium (long acting muscle relaxant) for maintaining relaxation when Suxamethonium wears out. After induction and intubation, I use the same 2ml syringe to draw 20 units Syntocinon (given for effective uterine contraction immediately after delivery to push the placenta out, as well as to minimize postpartum bleeding). Then I use the same 2ml syringe for Fentanyl, a narcotic supplement. Until then, anesthesia is maintained with Nitrous Oxide, Oxygen and very low concentration of Halothane. Normally, up to 8mg Vecuronium will be required to maintain muscle relaxation for Cesarean sections lasting up to an hour. Since it was likely to be a vaginal delivery and not expected to take more than fifteen minutes, I casually picked another 2 ml syringe to draw just half the dose of Vecuronium instead of the 5ml syringe and kept it separately. I have never done this before and never since. As no other trained person was available to resuscitate the infants, I planned things in such a way that I would be free to deal with the twins the moment they arrived, leaving the mother secured to a mechanical ventilator with a longer acting relaxant.

In this horrifying instance, I grabbed the wrong 2ml syringe by mistake and injected the full dose of Syntocinon instead of Vecuronium when the Suxamethonium wore out. I was aghast and was just too late to realize that I had in fact given 20 units of Syntocinon. I still had to give Vecuronium as well to settle the patient. This mix-up had never happened to me in my entire career and was unforgivable. The 20 units of Syntocinon would bring about a powerful and sustained uterine contraction within a minute of administration and kill the twin fetuses, which were already distressed. It was a genuine mistake in a situation where I had to handle several matters simultaneously. I was deeply remorseful and totally helpless. The obstetrician had just donned his gown and gloves, and the patient was already positioned for manual vaginal delivery. I remained stone silent and could think only of my preceptor and savior, Bhagavan Baba, who had in the past saved me from many impossible situations. In desperation, I prayed for instant help. Outwardly I pretended to be calm as if all was well. My thoughts drifted in the next couple of minutes as follows:

"Swami! Please forgive me for this. I was called to help save the twins and, instead, I have given them the fatal blow. How can I face the world, the profession and the mother in particular, who will be so distraught, especially since this is her first pregnancy? Before long I will face litigation and substantial claims for damages." So dejected, I concluded this would be my last anesthetic in this life. "Any minute the obstetrician is going to yell at me, 'What have you done?' as he discovers the uterus contracted hard as rock." My reverie concluded but nothing happened. I was surprised by the silence. The obstetrician proceeded vigorously with his job, his entire hand inside the uterus trying to grab hold of the leg of the first twin. I couldn't believe my eyes. I asked him if all was well at his end, and he replied, "The uterus is relaxed, and I have got hold of one leg. It will be a vaginal delivery," he confirmed much to my relief. A feeling of intense gratitude to Swami, my Almighty, overwhelmed me.

Before long, the first twin was delivered and came out screaming. Within three minutes, the second twin did the same. There was no need whatsoever for me to do anything for the infants. The midwife and the junior nurse attended to them. As soon as the second twin was out, the obstetrician asked me to give 20 units Syntocinon. I did not give any further dose of the drug, the first dose having been wrongfully given 10 minutes earlier. I paused for a moment talking to Swami within: "You, who had the power to stop the action of this drug 10 minutes ago can also release the brakes now and let the uterus contract". I told the obstetrician, "20 units given." After 90 seconds, I asked him if the contraction was satisfactory, and the one word answer was "fine." What grace! What an incredible experience for me witnessing His divine power, not just over the elements of nature, but manifesting beyond time and space. Where and how was my thought linked to His mighty will? Where does this leave our limited science?

I did not reveal this mind-boggling experience right away to anyone with the exception of the immediate members of my family and a few close Sai devotees. In due course, I did narrate this inexplicable event to some of my colleagues. Some of them believed me as they knew my straightforwardness, but they were dumfounded. Others tried to persuade me to accept that I had imagined that I had administered the wrong drug but, in fact, had given the correct one. "How come then," I asked, "didn't I have to inject the contents of the second syringe to settle the patient? Ten minutes later, with no drug yet given, and as soon as I had the mental connection with Baba, the uterus contracted firmly." Because I had worked with this particular obstetrician for over fifteen years, and he respected my integrity, I decided, a few years later, to narrate this hair-raising experience to him. He listened to the entire story with awe.

The Dead Fetus Lives

The birth of our first grandchild in 1992 was nothing but high drama. At twenty-eight weeks, our elder daughter went into premature labor on the eve of her Part I Anesthesia examination and was admitted to the hospital. In the delivery suite, intravenous medications were administered to avert a very premature delivery. Vibhuti was applied to the abdomen, and our prayers were answered in twenty-four hours when contractions began to abate. After forty-eight hours, she was transferred to a private room for a week of bed rest before being discharged. At thirty-two weeks, she was again hospitalized for bed rest for severe Pregnancy Induced Hypertension (PIH). Hypertension and generalized edema persisted even after treatment. Ultrasound scan and amniocentesis for hormonal assay (L/S ratio) were done at thirty-five weeks to check fetal viability. For the safety of mother and to salvage the infant, they decided to induce delivery forthwith and not wait any longer.

Early the next morning, membranes were ruptured and Syntocinon infusion commenced to induce labor. For some mysterious reason, the fetus reacted badly to Syntocinon, and the fetal heart stopped as evinced by the fetal tachograph tracing and confirmed by absent fetal heart sounds on auscultation. An urgent Cesarean section was indicated. As no one else was around, I was asked to anesthetize my daughter, and my son-in-law, who was also a physician, was asked to assist with the operation. It still took more than twenty minutes to have the operating room ready. Within two minutes from induction of anesthesia, a lifeless baby boy was delivered. I could not attend to the baby until I secured the mother's safety. The baby was tiny, bluish-gray and not breathing. There were no heart sounds either. Thirty minutes had elapsed since the heart stopped in the womb, and the infant was delivered dead. There were no extra hands to help us. I left the mother in the care of a mechanical ventilator and did my best to resuscitate the infant knowing it was an impossible task. Using an infant Ambu resuscitator, I gave external cardiac massage with my left hand and pushed some oxygen into the lungs with the other. I called on Swami for help, praying for the baby not to have any brain damage if it ever pulled through. At best I managed to get the heart beat up to 70 per minute from naught. The rate should be over 140 for a normal infant. The little one was just gasping without much improvement in color. I peeked outside the door and asked my wife and younger daughter to send the SOS to Swami.

We decided to sedate our daughter heavily for twenty-four hours, because we knew she would be unduly distressed about the fate of her precious son. We were not sure how long the baby might last. No one there even knew how to operate the controls of the brand new Intensive Care crib, one of the latest models and highly technical. "Sai Ram" was the only magic word on all our lips. While the mother was "bombed out" with heavy sedation, others awaited a miracle or the inevitable. A pediatrician arrived later and got the crib working. It was too late even to consider transferring the baby to a high-tech neonatal ICU. We left it all in the divine hands. My son-in-law went home and prayed, lighting an incense stick in the prayer room. Baba responded with His presence and reassurance evinced by the ash from the burnt incense remaining stiff, without falling, in the shape of the letter 'S'! Now and then, we could smell whiffs of jasmine around the crib too. The first eighteen hours were a nightmare for all of us.

Overnight, some mysterious hand pulled out the infant feeding tube. When I dropped in at 5:00 a..m., the baby was still not moving its limbs. Although the nurse was upset, I felt that the feeding tube coming out might be a divine sign that the baby could be taken to the mother's bosom. The infant surprised us all by feeding like it was a normal baby. The merciful Lord had turned things around. What grace! Then, as the 2.2kg baby steadily improved, so did the mother with her hypertension clearing. On the fifth day all were home. We still needed Baba's continuous "presence" around the infant and for months, around the clock, played the CD with His melodious chanting of the Gayatri Mantra in the baby's bedroom. The following week, I visited Sai Baba and thanked Him for the gift of life to our grandson. Swami named the boy Adithya, meaning sun. Yes, through Adithya, He has filled us with the warmth of love and the light of wisdom.

Our Move to Prasanthi Nilayam

In July 1992, the call came for me to settle in Prasanthi Nilayam and serve Sai Baba in the Super Specialty Hospital. I had to delay my preliminary visit because of the complications related to our daughter's pregnancy. Our relationship with Baba, at the physical level, periodically swings from close interaction and interviews to being distanced or kept in cold storage. We had been in cold storage since 1988. The thaw began with three consecutive dreams around Guru Pournima in 1992. The first dream was on the night prior to Guru Pournima. The place was something like St. Peter's square at the Vatican. Baba was supposed to be on the fourth floor locked in with a few close devotees. I was one among thousands waiting for the doors to open to have a glimpse of Baba. I felt I had waited long enough and started scaling the vertical wall, risking a fatal fall. Somehow

I managed to roll over the baluster railing onto the fourth floor balcony and enter a large hall where Baba was in the midst of several of His devotees. When Swami saw me, He walked towards me, and I rushed towards Him and bowed at His feet. As my head touched his feet I clearly heard Him say inside my head, "If you walk in front of Me, don't expect Me to follow you. If you walk behind Me, you may lose Me. Learn to walk with Me, and I will walk with you." Giving me a warm welcoming smile, He permitted me to stay with Him. With this dream, He gave me the first sign that the turn around was imminent.

The second dream was on the very next night, the night of the auspicious Guru Pournima. In this dream I was administering anesthetic to a child in Room 1 of the Urology OT complex. Baba walked up to the large glass door and blessed us raising His right hand. I had never seen the hospital, let alone the layout of the Urology OT. This turned out to be an actual preview of exactly what happened when Baba visited the hospital on December 30, 1993. I had started working there only a few weeks earlier. With this dream, He confirmed that I would be appointed to the Super Specialty Hospital just as He had predicted twelve years earlier on December 29, 1980. The third dream was on the night after Guru Pournima. Baba was in the midst of His guests, and He was telling them something as He pointed towards me. Since taking up residence in Prasanthi Nilayam, I have seen Swami do exactly this when He was introducing me or His senior staff to visiting dignitaries.

While I was having these dreams in Sydney, Swami was speaking to Sri V. K. Narasimhan, editor of the *Sanathana Sarathi* (a monthly Sai magazine*)*, telling him that my wife and I should wind up our affairs in Sydney to come over and serve in His hospitals. A few weeks later, Mr. Narasimhan's son, Mr. Prahalad, was visiting his daughter in Sydney and personally brought me this message from his father. This confirmed my dreams. Although I visited Swami at the end of September 1992 to finalize our move, it was not until November the following year that we were able to leave Sydney according to Swami's directive. We have now completed seven years of residence in

Prasanthi Nilayam and feel so blessed to have the opportunity to serve in Baba's hospitals.

Unlike in western countries, where I had practiced most of my life, we work six days a week here. Because I was not used to this, in the beginning I found it difficult to adjust to the six-day schedule. The workload is heavy, and the hours we spend in the operating theaters can be long. Baba says, *Work is worship; Duty is God.* It has taken many years to get over this mental block and be able to transform work into worship. Swami also says, *Hands that serve are holier than lips that pray.* Without constantly remembering all this, it is not too difficult to get caught up in the old habits and feel exhausted or depressed. To live with joy in this new paradigm becomes easy if we can understand and experience the wholesome spiritual value of selfless love and service. To be at peace and be fulfilled through work, as service to God, is a great learning process. This is especially so in the midst of many challenging situations. Swami has blessed me with some inspirational wisdom, and often I get ideas—such as what follows—which can bring better understanding among the operating room personnel.

"The operating room personnel should be like a family living in harmony. The surgeon, like the husband, is the head of the family. The anesthetist, like the wife, is the sheet anchor for the operating room stability. The nurses are like close relatives, without whose goodwill and cooperation the operating theaters would come to a halt. The technical officers are like friends, and the cleaners are like the domestic servants. Just as all of the household work together for the welfare of the children, all OT personnel must do their part and work in harmony and understanding for the welfare of patients, who are like children and totally dependent on us. When there is rivalry between the husband and wife and ego reins supreme, the children suffer. Likewise, if there is no mutual respect but a power struggle between the surgeon and the anesthetist, the patients suffer. The anesthetist plays a leading role in the efficient running of the operating room just as a housewife, whose invaluable input, makes a house a livable home."

Thus, the anesthetist can play a pro-active and pivotal role in the smooth running of the operating theaters. Benefits are enormous when we spiritualize the atmosphere in the operating room. By working in awareness of reality and drawing inspiration, guidance and help from the infinite source, we bring good and wholesome results. I have experienced this and am personally aware of this power at work in the operating room. A few of my colleagues in Australia, and several of them over here in Baba's specialty hospital, recognize this as well. Sometimes after a procedure, my colleagues in Australia would ask me what made the difference. My answer has always been simple. I tell them that I prayed for help, and my preceptor and master in India, Sai Baba, was helping us. Indeed, a couple of eminent surgeons in Sydney, one a professor of surgery and the other a professor of orthopedics, have openly asked me to pray to Sai Baba in the middle of operations for help in crisis situations. Several times, our gracious Lord has responded to our prayers.

Sai-chiatric Shock, Not Psychiatric Shock

In March 1995, before we left Prasanthi Nilayam on our annual visit to our family in Australia, Swami gave us two of His robes, one for our Sai Center in Sydney and the other for our personal use. Within a day of our arrival in Sydney, I received a phone call from a friend of ours who sounded desperate. He said, "I am pleased you are back from India. We are facing a serious crisis in the family. I am calling you, because I believe you can help us out of our dire situation." Not knowing what the crisis was about, I replied, "With Sai Baba's help and your belief, I will do whatever I can. It will be as the Lord wills and if He lets me be His instrument. Tell me, what's so desperate?"

He told me that the crisis was about their sixteen-year-old son who was threatening to commit suicide. His eldest son, Joe, had been in the children's psychiatric wing of a leading teaching hospital in Sydney for seven weeks. He was about to be transferred to Redbank House at Westmead, a brand-new high-security unit purposefully built to deal with high-risk cases, especially teenage suicide. No longer interested in life, Joe had attempted suicide twice, once in hospital custody while on medication. Australia ranks high in the world for teenage suicides. He was an eleventh year student attending a good private school and doing very well in studies, music and sports. At the request of his parents, the hospital reluctantly agreed to delay his transfer until I visited him. I am neither a psychiatrist nor a counselor, only my faith in Baba gave me confidence. I left everything in Baba's hands. Armed with Baba's robe, I dashed across the city to meet Joe, who was waiting in an office room under the care of a welfare worker who was to accompany him to Redbank House. Joe did not know why their journey was delayed and was surprised to see me.

I had known this boy from his childhood and had even given him anesthetic twice for ear surgery. The family are Catholics but well aware of Sai Baba and knew why we visited Him. While Joe was happy to see me, he was also suspicious because his parents had sent me to see him. At that time, he had some resentment towards them. I gave him Baba's robe to hold while we talked. He could not believe that he was actually holding a robe Baba had worn. I tried to convince Joe that I had loved him from his childhood and that I had come to see him in the names of Christ and Sai Baba, not for his parent's sake. Although not entirely convinced, he chose to remain neutral towards me and did not mind my visiting him again at Redbank. I was happy we had an entirely private session, lasting almost an hour, while the welfare officer waited outside.

Joe did not want his parents to visit him at Redbank. The authorities agreed to permit me to visit him as requested by his parents, and I visited Joe almost every evening after work. Our conversations were general. Joe was on heavy doses of anti-depressants, and they were planning to give him shock treatment (ECT) for which his parents refused to give consent. I learned from the nurse in charge that Joe was really looking forward to my visits. Whenever possible, I took some home-made food, which he ate with relish as it was a change from the bland hospital diet. Our relationship steadily improved, and Joe began to trust me. In the beginning, he was categorized as high risk and confined to a single room with one-to-one supervision including the use of a close circuit TV monitoring. Within a week, I noticed the nurse was happy to leave him alone and step out of the unit.

Something prompted me to take Baba's robe on my next visit. I hoped the nurse would go out for awhile, as usual, and no one would be there to keep watch over us. I asked Joe if he would like to meditate with me, and he agreed. I sat next to him on his bed and pulled out the robe and asked him to hug it. When I saw myself sitting right in front of a mirror over the washbasin across the bed, I was "prompted" to swap seats with him so that he could see himself in the mirror. I asked Joe to relax and keep looking into his eyes, not at his face or anything else. I kept repeating softly, "Into your eyes Joe... into your eyes." I am no hypnotist but have seen them at work in movies. After a few minutes, I also turned his focus to conscious breathing, all the time reminding him to keep looking into his eyes – "Into your eyes... into your eyes.... Breathe in... and breathe out..." I also reinforced the process with some Christian affirmations and the beauty of the real person within.

As Joe settled into this rhythm and kept his eyes focused, I asked him to continue with the mediation while I sat by his side quietly and prayed for him. Hardly two minutes had elapsed when he let out a hysterical scream and grabbed me. In self-defense I got a firm hold on him fearing the worst might happen. He was breathing heavily and, when he started releasing his grip, I realized that he had a fearful experience but now felt secure in my arms. Fortunately, none of the hospital staff was around which gave me a great sense of relief. I asked Joe what had happened.

Gasping he said, "Those eyes."

"What eyes?" I probed, and he repeated the same words.

When quizzed further he said, "That face."

"What face?" I asked.

"That hair... that face," he exclaimed.

"What hair are you talking about? Come on, tell me." I persisted, and he said nothing, still gasping with fear all over his face.

"I saw Him; I am scared..." he said.

"Whom did you see?" I demanded.

"Him…" was his response.

"Was it Sai Baba?" I asked. Joe nodded in the affirmative.

"You mean, you saw the face of Sai Baba? Where were you then?" I quizzed. He replied, "Only Him."

While I lovingly put my arm round his shoulders to help him overcome his stress, I clarified, "You disappeared and there was only Sai Baba in your place? What an experience! How lucky and blessed are you. Here I am, visiting Sai Baba every year, sometimes twice a year since 1980, and still struggling to experience this oneness. And without any effort you have experienced this great unity—you in Him, He in you, and the oneness of both. I am so happy for you Joe and, believe me, Sai Baba and Christ are one. What happened here is proof that Sai Baba will help you out of your impasse soon."

He was listening to every word I said while still not quite out of the shock. We relaxed for a while and later talked about his interests and things in general. He asked me when we were returning to Sai Baba. He told me that, although he was brought up a Catholic, he had never accepted Christ alone as the savior. He wanted to know more about Sai Baba and asked me if I would bring something about Sai Baba for him to read. We hugged each other before I departed. I also advised him not to tell anybody at Redbank about what had happened that day. When I visited him the next day, I gave him *Sai Baba, the Holy Man and the Psychiatrist* by Dr. Sandweiss. Joe was excited to see me, especially because he had dreamt of Sai Baba the previous night.

In his dream, Sai Baba had appeared at the door of his room and was holding an umbrella with a pointed shaft. Joe saw cut pieces of his body strewn across the floor of the room. Sai Baba walked into the room and poked the umbrella shaft into one of the pieces like a barbecue stick. Pointing it towards him, Baba told Joe, "I am taking this troublesome piece away from you, and you will be well once again," and walked away. "What an incredible dream," I thought, "and to take place on the same night as the startling experience during meditation." I came to know later that his mother also had a dream that same night, where she saw herself and Joe in a room with Sai Baba, and she was reverentially prostrating at His feet. Is this coincidence or divine reassurance?

Later, I drew Joe into a discussion on the significance of his dream. I asked him, "Who was that who saw, and whose body was cut into pieces on the floor? How did you know they were pieces of your body and not kangaroo meat?" Joe was nonplused but insisted that he knew that they were pieces of his body. He became confused when I had raised this query about his physical reality, because he had no doubt about seeing pieces of his own body. It was too much for the young man to comprehend consciousness at a higher astral level. I tried to explain to him that, in the dream, he had experienced his real Self who was not limited to the body and who had witnessed the body in pieces. I added that the dream was more than symbolic in that the causative factor that was responsible for his suicidal tendency had now been taken away by Baba and that he was well on the mend. Instead of electric shock (Psychiatric Shock), Baba had cured Joe using "Sai-chiatric" shock. We were overjoyed with the events of these two days. The doctors were surprised to see such a dramatic improvement in Joe. Two weeks later, he was discharged from Redbank. Since then, he has led a normal life, stopped all medications and continued with his education without interruption, securing a high mark and place for his desired course in the university.

Amazing Grace

Between June 1993 and September 1994, Swami repeatedly reassured Venkatesh, a long-standing devotee: *I shall look after everything.* He had also materialized vibhuti on several occasions, blessed a lingam and asked him to drink the lingam water. In September 1994, Swami asked Venkatesh to leave his job in Nigeria and come to Him. A week after his arrival, on October 1st, he had a massive heart attack while Swami was speaking during the evening session at Trayee Brindavan (Bhagavan's residence in Whitefield). Just before this, he suffered from profuse sweating and breathlessness and took vibhuti three times saying, "Sairama, Sairama, Sairama." Believing that Venkatesh had just fainted, the students splashed some water on his face to revive him. Swami, appearing quite unconcerned, continued with His talk while seated on the joula (ceremonial swing). Meanwhile, a doctor seated nearby examined Venkatesh and declared him dead. When the situation was conveyed to Swami, He abruptly stood up, picked up His silver cup containing water and walked towards Venkatesh's body that was lying flat on the floor. Venkatesh told us later that he had an out-of-body experience in which he had heard the sounds of gushing water while being driven into pure light. He saw his body lying horizontally on the floor with Baba standing next to it.

Swami poured water on His right hand and let it trickle over His thumb into Venkatesh's mouth. Then He commanded: *Your Sai-Rama has come. Get up.* After Swami had repeated this a few times, the inert body jerked and the eyes opened. Bringing him to life, Swami looked at the staff and told them, *What other miracle do you want? He was gone, and I brought him back.* The remaining session was canceled and Swami asked the staff to bring Venkatesh to His room. Bhagavan blessed him, and three other doctors also examined him. The ECG done the next morning showed an acute infarct. Baba was promptly informed and, for twenty days, He treated Venkatesh only with vibhuti, told him to rest and sent him for a check-up at the Super Specialty Hospital.

A few weeks later, Baba returned to Prasanthi Nilayam and continued treating Venkatesh until December 1994. Baba then gave Venkatesh permission to return to Nigeria telling him, *No medicine from now on.* Venkatesh did not take even an aspirin from then until July 1999.

I hardly knew Venkatesh until April 1999 when destiny brought us together. Towards the end of June, Venkatesh began complaining of tightness in the chest. One afternoon during darshan, Swami looked at Venkatesh and told him to get himself checked up at the hospital. A routine examination revealed significant myocardial ischemia. Venkatesh would not even take the prescribed angina tablets. He had complete faith in Swami and would only agree to an angiogram if Swami approved it. After keeping him waiting for five days, Swami told him to get the angiogram done. The angiogram showed three significant blockages and a CABG (Coronary Artery Bypass Graft) was indicated. Swami approved the operation and said He would fix the date for the operation. He surprised everyone by personally visiting the patient in the hospital, spending over twenty minutes showering His love as vast as the ocean and attending to every minute detail. Before He left the room, Bhagavan materialized vibhuti and even lifted His lotus feet up to the bed for Venkatesh to take padnamaskar. He assured him that He would take care of everything and that Dr. Voleti from the USA had been summoned to perform the operation. As soon as the surgeon arrived, Swami came to see Venkatesh and finalized all arrangements for the operation the following morning.

Overwhelmed by the unfolding events, Venkatesh spent a restless night before surgery and developed some chest pain. Although the operation was scheduled for 9:00 a.m., during the morning darshan, Swami asked the team to start the anesthetic by 7:30 a.m. It was clear that Swami knew what would happen, perhaps a fresh attack, necessitating a postponement. The operation was completed and the patient moved to the ICU and extubated sooner than usual. Swami's invisible hand at work was perceived by the manner in which some difficulties were overcome. The chest tubes are usually removed on the third postoperative day and, occasionally, some blood clots may dislodge and drop inside the chest cavity. Clearly this had happened, because Swami came in the patient's dream, pulled away the dressings and put His hand over the drainage site and pulled out some blood clots. This was repeated twice to ensure no clots were left behind. The rest of the hospital stay was uneventful, although the patient experienced the infinite love and "presence" of Swami in many ways.

The night before he left the hospital, Venkatesh had a dream in which Swami walked into his room, asked him to lift up his shirt and, pressing His ear against his chest, listened to his heart. Bhagavan declared that everything was perfect, and that he should go back to the ashram. During darshan the following morning, Swami instructed the surgeon to discharge Venkatesh from the hospital.

I consider myself extremely fortunate to have found my personal and loving God in Sri Sathya Sai Baba, whom countless millions throughout the world love, adore and worship. The homeward journey towards peace and fulfillment began with Sai Baba's entry into my life. Until then, God was merely a concept. I did not know who or what God was. Conventional beliefs and customs gave me no satisfaction. They only helped me to drift away from God. I badly needed to experience God to believe in Him—His love, splendor and supremacy. I was fortunate to seek Him at a time when my life was on a reckless course in the fast lane of modern materialism. I recognize there is the right time for everything, just as there is the right time for the butterfly to fly out from the chrysalis. Although it is said that God is omnipresent and omnipotent, until we experience this, these remain mere ideas. I have been fortunate to personally experience Him, as have the multitude of devotees from almost every country in the world. Yes, Baba has incarnated in the human form vested with all the powers of divinity. But because He is shrouded in maya, a rationalist cannot comprehend Him.

The heart alone will resonate with divine love. Love, devotion, and selfless service are the doorway to experience the divine mystery. Time and again, Sai Baba has demonstrated this by making impossible things possible. When Swami became the center of our lives in 1980, all other interests in life were instantly given up. Such an overnight change of priorities, without Sai's grace, was unthinkable. Shakespeare said, "There is a tide in the affairs of men, taken at flood will lead on to fortune; omitted, all the voyages of life may stagnate in shallows and misery." When the flood of grace overflowed, I wisely let my boat rise with the tide.

Love All, Serve All

GLOSSARY

Advaita: Non-dualism refers to the nature of reality, God; everything is God. All, the creator and creation, is One.

Akhanda Bhajan: 24 hours chanting for world peace and happiness.

Atma: The spark of God within, the soul.

Avatar: An incarnation of God; descent of God on earth for the upliftment of humanity.

Bhajan: Devotional song.

Bhagavan: The Lord; God.

Darshan: Seeing a holy person. To see the form of the Lord and receive his blessings.

Gayatri Mantra: Sacred chant that both protects and illumines the mind of those who recite it.

Gopis: Cowherd maids who worshipped Lord Krishna.

Guru Pournima/Gurupurnima: Hindu holiday set-aside for adoration of the guru.

Jai : Victory.

Japamala: 108 beads used in the repetition of the name of God or a mantra; similar to a rosary.

Krishna: Lord Krishna, an avatar who lived about 5000 years ago.

Leela: God's sport, God's divine play.

Mandap: An area facing the temple where devotees sit for darshan.

Mandir: Temple.

Maya: The deluding power of the divine which obscures the vision of God. The primary illusion is the world as perceived through the five senses.

Om: The most sacred word of the Vedas. The original first sound of the supreme universal reality called Brahman.

Padnamaskar: Touching the feet with devotion, symbolizing surrender to the Lord, and considered a great blessing.

Prasad: Blessed food.

Pranams: To bow in reverence.

Satsang: Gathering in the company of good people, usually spiritual aspirants.

Sai Gayatri: A special mantra given to one of Sai Baba's devotees. Gayatri means that which saves when repeated. The Sai refers to Sai Baba.

Sairam: Name for Sai Baba used as a greeting and unspoken prayer by his devotees. This Sai avatar is the same as the Rama avatar.

Seva: Selfless service as worship of the divine.

Seva dal: Service workers in the Sai Organization.

Shirdi Sai: The name that Sathya Sai Baba was called in his previous incarnation.

Shivaratri: Literally, "the night of Siva." A time of austerity and intensified spiritual practice on the night of the lunar calendar when the moon is smallest and furthest from the earth therefore enabling spiritual aspirants to steady their minds and achieve liberation.

Sita: One of the three Godheads of Indian scripture, the others being Vishnu and Brahma.

Vedas: Sacred scriptures of the Hindus.

Vibhuti: Holy ash with curative powers frequently materialized by Sai Baba.

Vinayaka: Leader of all. Name of Ganesha, the elephant-headed God; one who leads and is the remover of obstacles.

Yuga: Era or cycle.

Sai Baba Books from 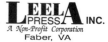 LEELA PRESS INC.

A Non-Profit Corporation
Faber, VA

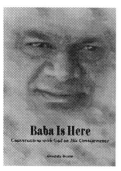

ISBN 1-887906-01-0
$12.00

Baba is Here by Graciela Busto. A beautiful example of how the Lord is omnipresent and available to all who seek Him. We are shown how we can find remarkable guidance by turning within. These inner dialogues with Sathya Sai Baba deal with the underlying nature of the universe and man's relationship to God. They explore the period prior to consciousness, providing detailed information about the purpose of life itself.

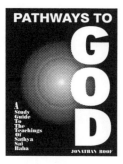

ISBN 0-9629835-0-0
$12.00

Pathways to God by Jonathan Roof. A clear and accurate guide to the teachings of Sathya Sai Baba. 27 chapters on topics such as peace, meditation and selfless service. Topics are presented and supported by numerous quotations from Sai Baba's writings.

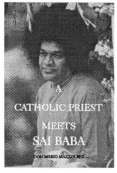

ISBN 0-9629835-1-9
$12.00

A Catholic Priest Meets Sai Baba by Don Mario Mazzoleni. A Roman Catholic priest, using his theological training, carefully examines Sai Baba's teachings and miracles. Finally, after nine visits to Sai Baba, his doubts dissolve as he sees how Baba's unconditional love and teachings mirror those of Jesus Christ. He asks, *Why would God limit Himself to incarnating only one time?* Through his meticulous investigation, and by direct experience, he realizes that Sai Baba is God alive in India today.

Sai Baba Books from LEELA PRESS INC.

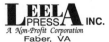

A Non-Profit Corporation
Faber, VA

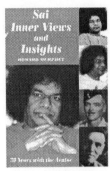

ISBN 1-887906-00-2
$12.00

Sai Inner Views and Insights *by Howard Murphet.* A compelling book by one of the world's greatest storytellers. Murphet traces his experiences with Sathya Sai Baba over the past 30 years. Not only does he describe miracles vividly, but he shares his experiences and insights into Sai Baba's teachings.

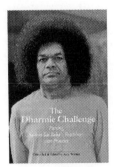

ISBN 0-9629835-6-X
$12.00

The Dharmic Challenge *by Judy Warner.* A provocative collection of stories that illustrate the difficulties of living a dharmic life. 14 Sai devotees explore different facets of dharma, such as Truth, Right Conduct, Duty and the need to be guided by conscience.

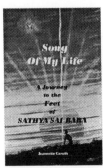

ISBN 0-9629835-8-6
$9.00

Song of My Life *by Jeannette Caruth.* A joyous and triumphant prose poem that gives the reader a vivid glimpse of the author's devotion and powerful insights into the nature of God. V.K. Narasimhan says, *No one can go through this poetic saga without feeling the thrill of a journey to God in the company of a devotee immersed in Divine Bliss.*

Sai Baba Books from LEELA PRESS INC.

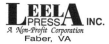

A Non-Profit Corporation
Faber, VA

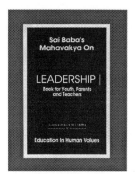

ISBN 0-9629835-4-3
$12.00

__Sai Baba's Mahavakya on Leadership__ by Lieut Gen (Retd) Dr. M. L. Chibber provides a blueprint for society on how to re-establish leadership inspired by idealism. A model for leadership appealing to everyone from corporate planners to government policy makers, to youth, parents and teachers.

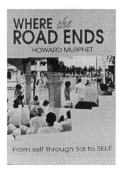

ISBN 0-9629835-3-5
$12.50

__Where the Road Ends__ by Howard Murphet. Murphet's personal search for the meaning of life from childhood to old age. *After I came to Sai Baba, He gradually revealed Himself to me as God. This book attempts to show how He brings greater and deeper understanding of life's purpose and a higher degree of happiness to the individual and thereby to the life of mankind.*

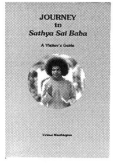

ISBN 0-9629835-2-7
$7.00

__Journey to Sathya Sai Baba, A Visitor's Guide__ by Valmai Worthington. A definitive guide for first time travelers to Prasanthi Nilayam. Written by an experienced Sai Baba group leader who shares the knowledge she has gained from helping hundreds of people over the last twelve years. This guidebook goes beyond providing answers to practical questions such as accommodations, food, dress and passports. It covers customs, behavior, and the subtle issues of readiness and spiritual awakening.

Brief History

Leela Press, Inc. was established in 1991 as a small non-profit company devoted to publishing books about Bhagavan Sri Sathya Sai Baba. To date, *Leela Press* has published fourteen books. Currently, ten are in print and available. *Leela Press* books are distributed worldwide. They are dedicated with love and devotion to Sathya Sai Baba.

~

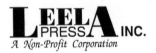
LEELA PRESS INC.
A Non-Profit Corporation

4026 River Road, Faber, VA 22938
Tel: (804) 361-1132 Fax: (804) 361-9199
email: jscher@leelapress.com